Report Writing for Speech–Language Pathologists and Audiologists

Report Writing for Speech–Language Pathologists and Audiologists

SECOND EDITION

Mary Pannbacker
Grace Middleton
Gay T. Vekovius
Kathryn L. Sanders

Contributions from
Merrie Pendergrass

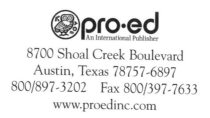
pro·ed
An International Publisher

8700 Shoal Creek Boulevard
Austin, Texas 78757-6897
800/897-3202   Fax 800/397-7633
www.proedinc.com

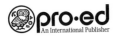

© 2001 by PRO-ED, Inc.
8700 Shoal Creek Boulevard
Austin, Texas 78757-6897
800/897-3202   Fax 800/397-7633
www.proedinc.com

Library of Congress Cataloging-in-Publication Data

Report writing for speech–language pathologists and audiologists / Mary Pannbacker . . .
   [et al.].—2nd ed.
      p.   cm.
   Includes bibliographical references and index.
   ISBN-13: 978-0890798676
   ISBN-10: 0-89079-867-2 (alk. paper)
   1. Speech therapy.   2. Report writing.   3. Medical writing.   I. Pannbacker, Mary H.
[DNLM: 1. Writing.   2. Ethics, Medical.   3. Medical Records.   4. Speech–Language
Pathology—methods. WZ 345 R425 2001]   00-045801
RC428.5 .R46   2001   CIP
808'.066616—dc21

This book is designed in Goudy.

Printed in the United States of America

5   6   7   8   9   10   10   09   08   07

To Robert Tate Wolcott
February 12, 1971–September 12, 1997

I know we will meet again sometime in the future. Be on the look out for me. I am the ray of sunshine through the trees, the birdsong in the forest, rain after a drought, the warm feeling of love. Now and then think of me and smile. I love you, Rob.

His passion was providing affordable, quality health care in health professional shortage areas.

Contents

Ethical Considerations in Report Writing

CHAPTER 1

Report writing is one of the responsibilities that audiologists and speech–language pathologists must discharge in an ethical manner (Knepflar, 1976). Ethical principles are voluntary or self-imposed disciplinary standards of professional practice for consumer protection (Flower, 1984). Ethical issues have been of concern to the American Speech-Language-Hearing Association (ASHA) since its founding in 1925 (Silverman, 1999). In fact, one of the reasons for founding ASHA was "to establish scientific standards and codes of ethics" (Paden, 1970, p. 73). All ASHA members and all holders of the ASHA Certificate of Clinical Competence must subscribe to the Code of Ethics. The purpose of this chapter is to discuss some of the ethical issues involved in report writing.

ASHA's Code of Ethics

The ASHA Code of Ethics (ASHA, 1994a) contains several statements related to report writing. These concern negligence and malpractice, nondiscrimination and the right to services, confidentiality, professional qualifications, advertising and public information, plagiarism, inaccurate reporting of results, objectivity, intra- and interprofessional relationships, and misrepresentation.

Negligence and Malpractice

Negligence and malpractice are legal rather than ethical issues, although these issues do involve some ethical constraints as well (Flower, 1984). ASHA's (1994a) Code of Ethics addressed these concerns: "Individuals shall hold paramount the welfare of persons served professionally. Individuals shall use every resource available including referral to other specialists as needed to provide the best service possible. Individuals shall evaluate services rendered to determine effectiveness . . . and shall provide services . . . only when benefit can reasonably be expected. Individuals shall not guarantee the results of any treatment or procedure directly or by implication; however, they may make a reasonable statement of prognosis" (p. 1).

The precept of "holding paramount the welfare of persons served professionally" implies that the clinician will use the most effective strategies available (Silverman, 1983). This precept, by implication, places several obligations on clinicians. First is an obligation to keep up to date by reading professional journals, attending workshops and conventions, and taking continuing education courses. A second obligation is to evaluate clinical strategies to determine effectiveness. Third is the obligation to advance clinical knowledge and techniques.

Although it might be hoped that all audiologists and speech–language pathologists would always provide services of exceptional quality, reality falls considerably short of that mark (Flower, 1984). At times, the shortcomings are so great that those services are clearly unacceptable or even harmful. Even when the overall quality of service is acceptable, errors may occur, with deleterious results. Lynch (1986) identified some potential sources of harm related to assessment procedures and misdiagnosis (see Tables 1.1 and 1.2).

Nondiscrimination and the Right to Receive Services

Most professional codes of ethics now include statements about nondiscrimination and the right to receive services. ASHA's Code of Ethics (1994a) contains the following statement: "Individuals shall not discriminate in the delivery of professional services on the basis of ethnicity, gender, age, religion, national origin, sexual orientation, or disability" (p. 1). Speech–language pathologists and audiologists are ethically bound to treat patients with HIV and AIDS. Clinicians who are pregnant have good reason not to work with patients who have HIV or AIDS because many patients with AIDS are infected with cytomegalovirus (CMV), a highly contagious disease that is dangerous in pregnancy and can result in congenital auditory defects and delayed cognitive development. It can be spread through contact with the saliva, urine, or feces of an individual carrying the disease (Kemp, Roeser, Pearson, & Ballachanda, 1995). Some patients with AIDS have not yet been diagnosed with CMV, so the clinician who is pregnant would be wise to avoid treating them (Brecker, 1993).

Table 1.1
Risks from Assessment Procedures and Errors of Omission

Error	Result
Improper placing, adjusting, or monitoring of oral prostheses such as palatal lifts or obturators	Tissue breakdown secondary to pressure; or the device could weaken over time, break, and fall into the airway
Improperly inserting speaking devices for patients on a respirator	Reduction in airflow
Incorrectly choosing augmentative devices for nonoral communication	If choice is below the client's abilities: Limitation of communication competence
	If choice is above the client's abilities: Frustration, withdrawal, decreased motivation to attempt communication or rejection of subsequent devices
Overlooking vocal changes or disregarding client's complaints of hoarseness and/or pain	Failure to identify symptoms of conditions such as cancer, papillomas, or vocal nodules needing medical treatment
Overlooking significant changes in speech or language skills in adults with aphasia or motor speech disorders	Life-threatening or medically treatable condition would go undetected
Improperly inserting objects in the ear such as ear molds, impedance probes, or probe tube microphones	Damage to the ear canal and tympanic membrane
Incorrectly using impedance in an ear with an open tympanic membrane and a perilymphatic fistula	Inaccurate test results leading to misdiagnosis
	Meningitis, possible death
Failing to use properly calibrated audiometric equipment	Incorrect test results leading to inappropriate treatment decisions such as a hearing aid when one is not needed
Overlooking important diagnostic indicators of acoustic neuroma or middle-ear pathology	Lack of medical referral and appropriate medical treatment

Note. From "Harm to the Public: Is It Real?" by C. Lynch, 1986, *Asha, 28*(6), pp. 28–29. Copyright 1986 by *Asha.* Reprinted with permission.

Table 1.2
Risks Secondary to Misdiagnosis

Delay in obtaining medical treatment
Emotional distress due to inflated or inaccurate prognosis
Inappropriate and/or unnecessary treatment decisions
Inappropriate educational and/or vocational recommendations
Increased delay in the development of speech and language skills
Increased severity because of delay in receiving appropriate services
Increased treatment time and increased expense due to lack of early intervention
Unnecessary financial expense
Unnecessary surgery

Note. From "Harm to the Public: Is It Real?" by C. Lynch, 1986, *Asha, 28*(6), p. 29. Copyright 1986 by *Asha.* Reprinted with permission.

Confidentiality

Reports contain confidential information and cannot be released without the written consent of the client or a responsible adult. Confidentiality applies to both oral and written communication between client and clinician and includes reports and other clinical records (Silverman, 1999). Information in a client's folder or computer database files is confidential; ordinarily it would be regarded as unethical to release the information without a client's permission. Individuals must not reveal to unauthorized persons any professional or personal information obtained from the person served professionally, unless required to do so by law or unless it is necessary to protect the welfare of the person or the community.

Clients and parents have a legal right (P.L. 92-380, Family Educational Rights and Privacy of 1974) to see any report containing information about them; thus, it is often useful to send them copies of reports (Emerick & Haynes, 1986). Generally, it is the legal guardian who gives consent to release confidential information, but in some cases consent from the guardian is not sufficient. For example, despite their legal incapacity, clients who are 16 or 17 years of age should be consulted regarding their willingness to have reports containing information about them released. In fact, younger clients may have definite opinions on whether or not they want reports released. Thus, a single source of consent may be necessary but not sufficient (Drew & Hardman, 1985).

Electronic information storage and transmission systems have created risks to confidentiality of information. Kuster (1997) described e-mail as "sending postcards where anyone between sender and receiver can read the message" (p. 33). Clinicians should inform clients about confidentiality issues related to e-mail (Landsman, 1999). In some situations, office staff intercept e-mail inquiries or companies reserve the right to check their employees' e-mail.

There are other issues related to confidentiality of client information, such as protection and security of computer-generated reports. These reports must not violate confidentiality regulations (Cornett & Chabon, 1988; Larkins, 1987). Chial (1984) pointed out that "if several users share secondary memory resources, 'privileged' information may be compromised" (p. 99).

Speech–language pathologists and audiologists should be familiar with techniques to safeguard confidentiality of electronic data, especially that which concerns clients (Probst, 1998; Scott, 1997). Passwords and access codes should serve as locked doors. In some instances, multiple password levels may be necessary for protection of client information. Other safeguards for confidentiality are listed in Table 1.3.

Clinicians should also be aware of changes in health care that have modified the traditional concepts of ethics (O'Neil-Pirozzi, 2001). These changes have occurred for several reasons: (a) the number of individuals involved in any single patient's care, indirectly and/or directly, has increased over time, making confidentiality more difficult to maintain; (b) patients' health care providers do not always have the same view of protecting confidentiality; (c) there seem to be discrepancies between what people feel they should do ethically and what they would do; and (d) the frequency that maintaining patient confidentiality conflicts with the law or would result in harm to the patient or others has increased.

Table 1.3
Strategies for Minimizing Confidentiality Risks

Implement audit trail to produce logs when files have been accessed.

Transmit only authorized data, not bulk photocopies or transmission.

Establish a unique patient identification system.

Strictly limit employees' ability to see individual employee medical/health records.

Discourage the sale of medical information to marketing firms.

Implement a procedure to identify duplicate or missing transmissions.

Develop procedures to verify the identities of those who request information.

Note. From "Protecting Patient Records," by M. A. Probst, 1998, *Advance for Speech–Language Pathologists and Audiologists.* Copyright 1998 by Merion Publications. Reprinted with permission.

Critical Review

Critical review of both published reports and clinical reports is an important ethical responsibility. Such review protects clients' welfare and provides assurance against unwarranted claims (Creaghead, 1999). Clinical decisions should be based on careful review of available information (Gillam, 1999). Some current strategies are considered by many to be fad treatments. These treatments are used by some clinicians but seriously questioned by others (Creaghead, 1999). Among them are treatments for central auditory processing disorders, temporal processing deficits, auditory integration training, sensory integration, and facilitated communication. Issues related to these treatment approaches were described in a series of articles in the October 1999 issue of *Language, Speech, and Hearing Services in Schools* (Duchan, 1999; Friel-Patti, 1999; Gillam, 1999; Griffer, 1999; Keith, 1999; Madell, 1999; Mauer, 1999; Tharpe, 1999; Veale, 1999).

Professional Qualifications

ASHA's Code of Ethics (1994a) addresses professional qualifications in the following ways: "Individuals shall honor their responsibility to achieve and maintain the highest level of professional competence. Individuals shall engage in the provision of services only when they hold the appropriate Certificate of Clinical Competence or when they are in the certification process and are supervised by an individual who holds the appropriate Certificate of Clinical Competence" (p. 2). Furthermore, "Individuals shall engage in only those aspects of the profession that are within the scope of their competence, considering their level of education, training and experience" and "Individuals shall continue their professional development throughout their careers" (p. 2).

Advertising and Public Information

ASHA (1994a) has included reference to advertising and public information in its Code of Ethics. "Individuals' statements to the public shall provide accurate information about the nature and management of communication disorders, about the profession and about professional services. Individuals must not misrepresent their credentials, education, training or experience. Individuals' statements to the public . . . shall not contain misrepresentations" (p. 21).

Misrepresentation of facts or deception of one type or another is an ethical issue. It refers to either an omission or a commission on the part of the clinician. A commission involves a situation in which the clinician gives false information. An omission means that the clinician simply did not inform clients about important aspects of the communication disorder, but withheld part or all of the information (Drew & Hardman, 1985).

Plagiarism

The ethical principles of scientific writing are designed to ensure the integrity of scientific knowledge and to protect the intellectual property rights of others (American Psychological Association, 1994). Writers must not present the work of another as if it were their own work. Credit must be given to another person or persons if their words or ideas are used. Reports submitted for academic or clinical course work must contain references and credit other individuals involved in the work (Hegde & Davis, 1999). For example, if two students collaborate in evaluating a client and writing the evaluation report, both students and the supervisor should sign the report. When reporting information described in a different report, the name of the clinician and the date of the report should be included. Plagiarism is failure to provide appropriate credit, and is considered to be illicit borrowing or stealing of someone else's ideas (Macrina, 1995). At best plagiarism is unethical, and at worst illegal (Bordens & Abbott, 1988). Plagiarism that is condoned, excused, or only lightly punished reduces individual and institutional integrity (Anderson, 1992). Principles of the ASHA Code of Ethics (ASHA, 1994a) specify "Individuals' statements to the public . . . shall adhere to prevailing professional standards and shall not contain misrepresentations" (p. 2). The revision of the ASHA (1999a) Code of Ethics proposed by the Board of Ethics states, "Individuals shall clearly reference the source when using other persons' ideas, research presentations, or products in written, oral, or any other media presentation or summary" (p. 5).

Inaccurate Reporting of Results

If speech–language pathologists or audiologists discover significant errors in their published data, reasonable steps should be taken to correct such errors in a correction, retraction, erratum, or other appropriate publication means. For example, there were errors in the speech sections of the *Journal of Speech, Language, and Hearing Research* (JSLHR) publications statistics for 1997 (Gordon-Salant, 1998). Corrected versions were published in the April 1999 issue of JSLHR (Metz, 1999).

Objectivity

ASHA's Code of Ethics (1994a) mandates that "Individuals shall maintain adequate records of professional services" (p. 1). Inadequate records accounted for several published violations of the ASHA Code of Ethics (Lass & Pannbacker, 1999). The need for maintaining objectivity is stipulated in the following principle: "Individuals shall not participate in professional activities that constitute a conflict of interest" (ASHA, 1994a, p. 2).

Various types of conflicts of interest exist. Ordinarily, discussion of conflicts of interest focuses on financial issues. Less attention has been given to intellectual conflict of interest, which is often elusive and difficult to define (C. R. King, McGuire, Longman, & Carroll-Johnson, 1997). C. R. King and associates (1997) indicate that "intellectual conflict of interest includes situations in which knowledge may contradict what is reported" (p. 166). For example, researchers may report only information that substantiates a view or position without providing information that does not support their contentions, or they may use their position to influence decisions.

Conflict of conscience is distinctly different from conflict of interest (Bradley, 1995). A conflict of conscience does not involve financial gain. It arises when the convictions of an individual override other considerations in reaching a decision. Speech–language pathologists and audiologists "must maintain objectivity in all professional activities, across all professional environments, and for all persons served" (ASHA, 1994b, p. 7).

Meitus (1983) indicated that "any piece of clinical writing should be a well-founded, objectively prepared document" (p. 299). Emerick and Haynes (1986) believe that "objectivity demands more than simple guarding against undue emotional involvement; the examiner must be objective about herself, her skills, knowledge, and personal characteristics" (p. 16). The two most frequently mentioned criteria used to determine objectivity are reliability and validity. Reliability is the consistency of a test or measurement procedure. Validity is the degree to which a test or measurement procedure measures what it is intended to measure (Maxwell & Satake, 1997; Polit & Hungler, 1991). The degree of objectivity differs. As objectivity increases, ambiguity and confusion decrease (Kerlinger, 1973). Lack of objectivity results in inaccuracies or errors that may range from minor, unintentional inaccuracies to outright falsification of information. The need for objectifying clinical reports has been emphasized by several authors (Darley, 1978a, 1978b; Emerick & Haynes, 1986; Mecham, 1979; Nation & Aram, 1977; Peterson & Marquardt, 1994; Silverman, 1985).

Intra- and Interprofessional Relationships

Ethical responsibilities related to intra- and interprofessional relationships are reflected in the following statements (ASHA, 1994a). "Individuals shall honor their responsibilities to the professions, and their relationships with colleagues, students, and members of allied professions. Individuals shall uphold the dignity and autonomy of the professions, maintain harmonious interprofessional relationships, and accept the professional self-imposed standards" (p. 2). It is interesting to note that Matkin, Ringel, and Snope (1983) reported that most of the 1,174 ASHA-certified audiologists and speech–language pathologists whom they surveyed rated their clinical competency relatively high in "communicating findings to others" and "collaborating with other professionals" (p. 97). Several studies have explored the opinions of other professionals regarding speech–language–hearing services (Moran & Pentz, 1987; Phelps & Koenigsknecht, 1977; Ruscello, Lass, Fritz, & Hug, 1980; Signoretti & Oratio, 1981; Tomes & Sanger, 1986). These studies indicated that other professionals generally have positive opinions about these services. In Table 1.4, good examples and

Table 1.4
Ethical Issues in Report Writing

Examples of Good Writing	Examples of Poor Writing	Explanation
Negligence and Malpractice		
"The hypernasality, nasal emission, and nasal grimacing suggest the need for direct, instrumental assessment of velopharyngeal function."	"Examination of oral structure and function revealed a short velum and velopharyngeal incompetence."	Do not hypothesize velopharyngeal incompetence in the absence of direct instrumental assessment.
"Radiographic and/or endoscopic evaluation of velopharyngeal function will be diagnostically beneficial."	"T and A is recommended for reduction of the hypernasality."	Do not make medical decisions.
"In view of John's age and stimulability, the prognosis for improvement is excellent."	"After a year of therapy, John's speech should be normal for his age."	Unreasonable/speculative statement of prognosis. This borders on promising a cure.
Description of nature and severity of speech–language problem.	"Diagnosis includes brain damage, mental retardation, or emotional maladjustment."	Do not make a medical or psychological diagnosis.
"John presented the following behaviors: self-stimulation, poor eye contact, and inappropriate laughter."	"The apparent autism has been unidentified by all the physicians who have seen John. Thus, it is recommended that they see Dr. Albert Jones, a competent psychologist, for an evaluation."	Do not criticize other professionals or make a referral to a specific person, unless that person is the only psychologist in town.
Nondiscrimination and the Right to Services		
Jane is a Native American.	"A Native American, Jane was neat and clean."	Avoid statements that suggest ethnic bias.
Information given in strictest confidence is not reported.	"The parents requested that information about an older sibling with multiple congenital malformations who died shortly after birth not be reported."	Do not report information given in strictest confidence.
Professional Competence		
"The purpose of the evaluation was to assess oral expressive language. The following tests were administered: *Test of Language Development–Primary, Structured Photographic Expressive Language Test, Expressive One-Word Picture Vocabulary Test.*"	"The purpose of the evaluation was to assess oral expressive language. The *Detroit Tests of Learning Aptitude* was administered."	Purpose and test protocol are inconsistent.
"John passed an audiometric screening."	"John had normal hearing on an audiometric screening."	Overgeneralization: Screening is either pass or fail.

poor examples of ethical issues related to report writing are provided with a brief explanation of each example. The information reported in the examples is fictitious.

Misrepresentation

The ASHA Code of Ethics (1994c) defines misrepresentation as "any untrue statement or statements that are likely to mislead. Misrepresentation also includes the failure to state any information that is material and that, in fairness, to be considered" (p. 1).

Wilkerson (2000) indentified misrepresentation in clinical reports as (a) extensive use of professional jargon; (b) reporting interpretations rather than observations; (c) indicating that a client did not perform a task that is very difficult than reporting a client could not perform a task; and (d) failure to provide sufficient facts to support a clinical conclusion. Wilkerson believes "failure to reliably identify and validly interpret clinical data may place the clinician at risk of violating ASHA's Code of Ethics" (p. 12).

Sanctions for Ethical Misconduct

Unfortunately, training and experience do not necessarily guarantee a high level of ethical integrity. Violations of ethical codes involve less rigorous consequences than do legal constraints (Flower, 1984). A code of ethics is adopted by an association and its members voluntarily subscribe to it. Thus, it exerts influence over only those professionals who belong to that association.

ASHA's Ethics Board (EB) (ASHA, 1992) is responsible for interpretation, administration, and enforcement of the Code of Ethics (ASHA, 1994a). Some of the penalties or sanctions for unethical conduct are to reprimand; censure; withhold, suspend, or revoke membership; or withhold, suspend, or revoke the Certificate(s) of Clinical Competence. EB decisions other than reprimand are published in *Asha* or more recently in *ASHA Leader*. A breach of ethics that is made public is embarrassing and causes professional disgrace. It may even cause one to lose a position (Drew & Hardman, 1985). The severest penalty is revocation of ASHA membership and certification, which essentially is expulsion from the profession.

Ethical Versus Legal Constraints

Flower (1984) and Green (1986) provided detailed discussions of ethical and legal considerations in audiology and speech–language pathology. Laws and codes of ethics may address similar issues; however, they apply different constraints. Laws and the regulations that elaborate those laws mandate specific qualifications for professional practice and define specific legal penalties for violations such as loss of the right to practice a profession, liability for fines, judgments requiring financial settlements, and loss of public funds to support professional services. Florida, in 1969, was the first state to enact legislation for licensing of audiologists and speech–language pathologists. All but three states, Idaho, Michigan and Vermont, and the District of Columbia now have enacted legislation for licensing of audiologists and speech–language pathologists (ASHA, 1997a; Rodgers et al., 2000).

Preferred Practice

Following the specifications and intent of the current ASHA (1994a) Code of Ethics, preferred practice patterns for audiology and speech–language pathology are strictly defined (ASHA 1997b, 1997c). The specific components related to documentation are as follows:

- Audiologists and speech–language pathologists prepare, sign, and maintain within an established time frame, documentation that reflects the nature of the professional service performed. When appropriate and with written consent, reports are distributed.

- Except for screenings, documentation addresses the type and severity of the disorder and any associated conditions (e.g., medical diagnosis, disability).

- Documentation includes results of previous related screening, assessment, and treatment procedures, if available.

- Results of assessment and treatment are reported to the patient/client and family/caregiver. (ASHA, 1997b, p. 10)

Summary

The principal goal of ethical standards is consumer protection. Ethical standards represent efforts toward professional self-regulation and provide detailed descriptions of self-regulation. These provide more detailed definitions of acceptable standards of professional practice than legal controls. Ethical integrity is mainly an individual undertaking. An important influence on ethical integrity is open discussion of professional ethics, problems, and potential outcomes of ethical misconduct (Flower, 1984; Green, 1986; Hanson, 1979; Jones, 1976; Knepflar, 1976; Pannbacker, Middleton, & Vekovius, 1996).

 Discussion Questions

1. Whom do audiologists and speech–language pathologists serve professionally?

2. How has electronic information storage and transmission created risks to confidentiality of information? How can these risks be reduced?

3. Why is critical review of information an important ethical responsibility?

4. How can plagiarism be avoided? Why should it be avoided?

5. What is an intellectual conflict of interest?

6. What is the difference between conflict of conscience and conflict of interest?

7. Describe ASHA's penalties or sanctions for unethical conduct.

8. What is the difference between ethical and legal sanctions?

Clinical Reports

Regardless of the professional work setting of the speech–language pathologist or audiologist (medical, public school, private practice, or community clinic), often the only communication medium reflecting a professional practice is in written reports. This may be somewhat unsettling to those who purposely chose a profession with a primary emphasis on oral communication or to those who labor at writing.

Many judge a clinician's professional/clinical competency based on written reports. Meitus (1983) feels that other "professionals will come to know and establish confidence in a clinician, in part, on the basis of what is committed to paper," and failure to write adequate reports diminishes "clinical effectiveness" (p. 290). Even minor errors in grammar and spelling may cause the reader to question the accuracy of the reported results, impressions, and recommendations (W. O. Haynes & Pindzola, 1998). R. King and Berger (1971) point out that "the efficiency of a clinic, school or agency can be evaluated by the thoroughness or lack of adequate reporting by its staff" (p. 113).

Standards for Reporting

Record keeping and the types of reports necessary to maintain a professional practice are specified in the standards (effective January 1, 1994) for Professional Service Programs Accreditation (ASHA, 1999f). The following indicators are the standards for maintaining client files:

- The program has a record keeping system for describing clinical activities, including communication about the client to and from other professionals, institutions, and programs.

- All records are organized with a consistent format and are legible, dated, and appropriately signed.

- Dated authorizations by the responsible individual (client, parent, guardian) are obtained for reports made to other professionals, institutions, and programs.

- Clinical reports contain information about the rationale, consistent with current knowledge about the disorder area, on which the clinical decision is based.

- In support of evaluation decisions regarding the diagnosis, impressions and recommendations, information about the tests and procedures used and the nature of the observations by the examiner and by other specialists are included. Consideration of the client's functional needs and cultural/linguistic environment should also be considered and included when appropriate.

- For treatment decisions, the nature of treatment procedures used and descriptions of obtained results are included based on the client's changing needs.

- Treatment plans include the type of services, frequency of the delivery of the services, and the probable duration of the speech–language pathology and audiology services without guaranteeing results.

- Clinical reports are disseminated within a specified time to appropriate persons and agencies.

- Policies and procedures for recording all clinical activities are evident.

- Screening activities are documented; hearing screening or a referral for an audiologic evaluation is included in all speech–language evaluations.

- Case records contain at least the following information:

    Client identification data

    Referral source and reason for the referral

    Pertinent information about the client such as medical records, psychological reports, educational tests, observations, and so forth.

    Name of speech–language pathologist or audiologist responsible for the evaluation

    Evaluation report(s) containing history information, summary of the examination results, and impressions and recommendations including a prognostic statement

Treatment plan(s) including specific objectives and prognostic statements

Chronological log of all services

Dated and signed information release forms

Progress reports, discharge summaries, and follow-up activities

Regardless of whether a program is Professional Services Board (PSB) accredited, procedures for documenting and tracking clinical reports and client files should be developed and strictly followed. Contents of reports should be in compliance with preferred practice patterns for the professions of speech–language pathology and audiology (ASHA, 1997b, 1997c).

Purposes for Reports

Reports are written in various forms and styles based upon their purpose, intended readers, and the preferences of the clinician or agency. The reason for writing influences what is written. The elements involved in writing complete a relationship among a reader, a writer, a text, and what is known about the subject matter. The purpose of clinical report writing is to inform the readers about something new to them. Thus, the writer must consider the literacy of parents and families as well as what the prospective readers already know about the subject. The term *clinical report* identifies the purpose of the report regardless of the targeted readers.

The major objectives of the diagnostic report are to

- provide a foundation or an entry point into the clinical service delivery system by providing baseline data or a record of conditions preceding management

- communicate specific findings about a client

- answer clinical questions such as whether the client has a problem and if so, whether treatment would be beneficial

- answer specific questions from referral sources or another professional

- act as a guide to referral for additional services

- provide documentation for accountability and quality assurance

- communicate information to and establish relationships with other professionals

- establish credibility of clinicians and their facilities

- teach the reader about communication disorders

- serve as documentation for research

- influence or persuade the reader to perform an action such as follow the recommendations stated in the report (Flower, 1984; W. O. Haynes & Pindzola, 1998; Knepflar, 1978; Lund & Duchan, 1988; Meitus, 1983)

The varying readers (physicians, parents, teachers, referring professionals, clients, etc.) determine the style of writing and amount of information included. Reports vary, and no single format is appropriate for all circumstances. In many instances, the format is determined by the clinical facility. For example, school clinicians report their findings in an Individualized Education Program (IEP). Clinicians in medical facilities report their diagnostic findings in the Problem Oriented Report (POR) or Subjective Objective Assessment Plan (SOAP) format. These formats are discussed later in this chapter.

Bangs (1982) believes that "reporting is an art and can be accomplished only by qualified examiners who are competent in reporting pertinent information to appropriate referral sources and who understand the feelings of parents who must receive the information" (p. 110). In addition to being competent and sensitive, the clinician must realize that information contained in a report represents an impression of a client obtained during a particular period of time in a given setting. It does not represent a complete picture of the client's communication ability. Furthermore, observation is no more accurate than the data upon which it is based. A written report based on observations of atypical behavior results in poor temporal reliability when the results from several sessions are compared. Thus, the writer must make clear that conclusions and recommendations are based upon history information, observations, and test results completed within the time frame of the evaluation.

Students and beginning professionals experience considerable stress and fear when assigned to write reports, particularly when they have inadequate training and experience. Baxley and Bowers (1991–1992) reported that students with more experience and training in writing reports had more positive attitudes about the process. However, students also reported that supervisors had differing standards or expectations when grading clinical reports, a condition that may contribute to increased stress about report writing.

Some seasoned professionals are poor writers. Those who write good clinical reports learned by having a "can do" and "will do" attitude about writing reports. They have studied the general principles of writing, identified and included all required elements of clinical reports, practiced revising and rewriting reports, and read and studied the reports written by others. Unfortunately, most have learned by trial and error because little attention has been given to teaching report writing. A time investment in teaching report writing is essential to improved writing and more positive attitudes about the process (Baxley & Bowers, 1991–1992). One cannot learn to write good reports by merely studying the writing process or by reading books about writing. Extensive practice with specific positive feedback on each practice attempt is needed to become a strong report writer (Hegde, 1998). Before practicing, however, one must have a working knowledge of the general principles of writing. Additional resources for learning about the writing process are available (Bates & Kromas, 1993; Berke, 1995; Blum, 1984; Elbow, 1998; Hegde, 1998; Kramer, Mead, & Leggett, 1995; Strunk & White, 1999; E. H. Weiss, 1990).

Principles of Writing

According to Knepflar (1978), it is "important that a system of report writing be developed whereby reports are concise, complete, well organized, and above all, honest" (p. 118). The information from the evaluation and interview is of limited value until it has been integrated in a clear, precise, efficient, and orderly format (Emerick & Haynes, 1986). W. O. Haynes and Pindzola (1998) add that a report should be made "alive" so that those who read it have a clear understanding of what occurred during the evaluation. This requires that notes recording all behaviors, impressions, and occurrences during the evaluation be taken quickly before the memory of the examiner fades. Most clinicians follow a busy daily schedule and see numerous clients. One cannot depend on memory to keep them all straight by the end of a busy day. Video and audio recordings are helpful aids to accurate reporting. Some agencies include in each file a photograph of the client.

To write a clear, concise, complete, well-organized, efficient, honest, and "alive" report, a clinician must study and practice language usage, report composition and form, and appropriate writing style. Basic rules for report writing are provided in Table 2.1 (Knepflar, 1976). Following these rules facilitates the development of a clear, understandable, accurate, grammatically correct, and succinctly written communication. Read through the examples of violations of the rules in Table 2.1 and rewrite them following the basic rules for effective writing.

The use of appropriate terminology is important to the accurate transmission of information. Table 2.2 provides appropriate and commonly used terms to identify the person receiving services, procedures used, professional completing the evaluation, and communication problems, as well as terms with a professional tone that identify or describe history information, observations, findings, procedures, and recommendations.

Being familiar with current terminology can be a professional challenge. Terminology changes over time. So-called buzzwords or politically correct terms tend to go in and out of style. Therefore, it is important to know the current preferred terminology of the populations served. Most important, the writer should keep the "person" foremost in the language (American Psychological Association [APA], 1994; Knepflar, 1976). Table 2.3 provides a summary of preferred terminology for reference to a client presenting problems other than or in addition to speech and language.

Diagnostic terminology tends to change. For example, attention deficit disorder would have been described as "distractible, hyperactive behaviors" in the 1960s. The use of preferred terminology for reporting a client's diagnosis is imperative. Neidecker and Blosser (1993) remind the writer to avoid emotionally charged words and phrases, which tend to promote hostility, guilt, fear, or suspicion in the reader. See Tables 2.3 and 2.4 for preferred terminology in reporting a client's diagnosis and describing observed behavior. Then rewrite the sentences in Worksheet 1.

The stated diagnosis when third-party payments are involved must conform to the terms used for speech, hearing, and language disorders in the *International Classification of Diseases–Ninth Edition* (ICD–9) (U.S. Department of Health and Human Services, 1994) and by ASHA (1997b, 1997c). Conditions are described by ICD–9 codes. Procedures are described by the Current Procedural Terminology (CPT) codes used for billing speech–language pathology and audiology services to Medicare, Medicaid, and private insurers. Reimbursement may depend upon the use of terminology for diagnosis. The clinician may not necessarily feel certain terms are most appropriate, but may need to use them nonetheless because that language is preferred by insurance carriers. In addition, coding for reimbursement can be confusing because the same regulations are interpreted differently by various programs, states, or insurance providers (Iskowitz, 1999). ICD–9 classifications that commonly pertain to speech, hearing, and language disorders are listed in Table 2.5. Procedure codes for speech–language pathology and audiology are found in ASHA publications (ASHA, 1997b, 1997c).

The composition and form of a report determine the way it reads. Ideally a report follows an orderly sequence in which the reader is guided through each major element and its supporting information. The report form or format determines the report writing style. Clinicians tend to develop a preferred report format and style; however, the agency or setting in which one works may adopt a uniform format developed to accommodate the limitations in writing time and secretarial support within the agency as well as the varied purposes of the reports. The report format used in hospitals is generally very different from that of speech–language–hearing clinics or schools. Most agencies develop a standard format for arranging the specific sections of their reports to assure continuity. Most clinicians adapt to the format provided in the work setting and continue to use a personal style of writing within that format.

Students in university training programs traditionally have not been taught to write the types of reports they will need to produce in varied off-campus practicum sites because of time constraints in the university curriculum and the tendency for reporting formats in medical, clinical, and school sites to be in a constant state of revision. Changes in federal and state laws and in medical reimbursement requirements are major reasons for modifying reporting practices in the various professional settings outside the university. In fact, increased productivity standards in rehabilitation settings have created frustration among speech–language pathologists because they have limited time to write abbreviated, quickly dashed-off reports and progress notes because this time is not "billable" (Hoolsema,

Table 2.1
Rules for Report Writing

Use	Avoid
Specific language	Ambiguous terms (example: "deafy speech")
Complete, clearly understood words	Abbreviations (example: "IMF positions" for "initial, medial, and final word positions")
Variety of language styles and words appropriate to needs of the report	Stereotypic or standardized language (unavoidable in checklist reports and some computer-generated reporting necessitating the importance of the "comments" section of such reports)
Specific, accurate, brief sentences	Verbosity and needless words (examples in Table 2.4)
Language that conveys sincere professional attitude	Flippancy (example: 5-year-old Shayla is a cute but ornery little dickens.)
Complete verb forms and correct punctuation	Contractions and hyphens (example: Joe's responses weren't consistent—not even in play.)
Positive statements that show what testing has revealed	Qualifiers and noncommittal language (example: Observations have revealed that Judy's responses were almost correct so these skills may possibly be emerging.)
Personal pronouns when they convey a clear statement in a natural manner	Awkward verbosity (example: Cathy's mother reported that she uses at least 50 words in conversation but her teacher says she uses about 20 words at school.)
Accurate descriptive language that is supported by fact	Exaggeration and overstatement (example: The client presents a fluency disorder that she will overcome with consistent environmental changes.)
The exact words to convey a concept or idea (consult a dictionary when in doubt)	Misusing words (example: David's stuttering is severe based upon the amount, type, and severity of his dysfluencies.)
Active verb construction when possible	Passive verb forms (example: Based on this examination, her speech and language skills were normal.)

Note. Adapted from *Report Writing in the Field of Communication Disorders*, by K. Knepflar, 1976, Danville, IL: Interstate Printers and Publishers.

1999). However, documentation is critical to whether services are reimbursed. Clinicians must provide extensive background information, long-term goals and objectives that can be readily quantified, and clear complete progress notes that substantiate the client's progress in meeting stated objectives. Reimbursement is more likely when notes are written in more detail, and insurance companies may be better informed about certain aspects of treatment based on clear, complete written documentation (Scott, 1998).

The clinician's documentation notes also serve to educate the Medicare provider. Thus, written evaluations, progress notes, and weekly summaries must be clear and complete. It is important that the clinician clearly describe treatment procedures and the client's response to them. Such documentation might include use of percentages, a description of the responses, and level of assistance needed to get the responses. Daily

notes are essential. Speech–language pathologists have an ethical responsibility to help patients access needed benefits. When denials for reimbursement are appealed, the best defense for funding is complete, accurate documentation. Such documentation may also contribute to future legislative reform (Crawford, 1998). The legislated Medicare Prospective Payment System (PPS) has created an environment in which less time can be devoted to documentation. Campbell (1999a, 1999b, 1999c) suggests that speech–language pathologists write less by documenting only the critical issues directly to the report form. Of course, this strategy saves time by eliminating the rough draft but increases the potential for writing errors. Many speech–language pathologists grieve their perceived loss of professional respect because the current medical environment offers so little time to write good reports (Hoolsema, 1999).

Table 2.2
Commonly Used Terms in Report Writing

Terms Referring to the Person Receiving Services

client, patient, child, youngster, student, the child's first name, Mr. or Ms. followed by surname

Terms Designating Clinical Activity Completed

treatment, remediation, intervention, speech rehabilitation, assessment, examination, testing, appraisal

Terms Referring to the Person Providing the Services

the (this) clinician, the (this) speech–language pathologist or therapist, the (this) examiner

Terms Identifying the Problems with Communication

Parameters Involved	*Identifying Terminology*
speech	abnormality
communication	anomaly
articulation	defect
language	deviancy
voice	deviation
rhythm	difficulty
fluency	disorder
hearing	dysfunction, impairment, problem

Professional Terms that Identify or Describe

ability, abilities	goal, goals	project, projects, projected
administer, administered	impression, impressions	reinforcement
appear, appears, appeared	improve, improves, improved	report, reports, reported
baseline	increase, increases, increased	respond, responds, responded
behavior, behaviors	indicate, indicates, indicated	response
carry over	informant, informants	reveal, reveals, revealed
causal	judgment	skill, skills
characteristics	nature	state, states, stated
conduct, conducted	objective, objectives	status
congenital	observation	symptom, symptoms
contingent	occur, occurs, occurred	symptomatology
criterion	onset	target behavior, behaviors
data	outlook	task, tasks
demonstrate, demonstrates, demonstrated	parameter	terminate, terminated
determine, determines, determined	perform, performs, performed	unremarkable
etiology, etiologies, etiological	performance	utterance, utterances
evidence, evidenced	produce, produces, produced	verbalize, verbalizes, verbalized
feedback	production	verbalization, verbalizations
generalize, generalizes, generalized	progressive	

Table 2.3
Preferred Terminologies

Preferred Terms	Terms To Avoid
persons who are disabled; people with disabilities; individuals who are physically challenged; individuals with physical involvement	the disabled; crippled; deformed; an invalid
congenital disability or involvement	defective at birth
partially sighted; visually impaired; blind (total loss of vision)	"blind" regardless of amount of vision; sightless
partial hearing loss; hearing impaired; deaf (total loss of hearing)	"deaf" regardless of amount of hearing; deaf-mute; deaf and dumb
Down syndrome	Mongoloid
mental or psychological disorder; mental illness	mentally defective; crazy; insane; deranged; demented; mad
learning differences	academic failure
person with mental retardation	retarded
nondisabled	able-bodied; normal
person with a seizure disorder	epileptic; victim of epilepsy
person with arthritis	arthritic; victim of arthritis
uses a wheelchair	confined to a wheelchair; wheelchair bound

Note. Adapted from "Reflections on Disability," by T. Carter, 1986, *Breakthrough.*

Students are generally taught a longer standard form of report writing so that they have experience writing history information, narrative descriptions of observed behaviors, specific explanations of tests and the client's performance on the tests, clear interpretation of the results included in the impressions along with prognostic statements, and complete and clear recommendations. With this experience, graduates should be able to adapt readily to abbreviated reporting formats in any professional setting. Students and professionals will find Reece's (1982) recommendations for composing readable reports helpful (see Table 2.6).

The style one uses for writing reports depends on individual preferences and the specific purpose or audience. Writing style is developed and becomes consistent and unique after repeated revisions. Andy Rooney (1986) asks, "When do I get good? How come what I wrote last year, last month, last week, and even yesterday, doesn't seem quite right, either?" (p. 11). Good writing takes practice. Speech–language pathologists often react with horror when they review a file completed in the past and notice glaring errors that were overlooked. It is realistic to view writing as a skill that requires continual refinement and active practice throughout one's professional career.

Common Errors and Exercises

When words are used incorrectly, confusion and misunderstanding may occur. Examples of commonly confused words are defined below and followed by practice activities.

Affect and *Effect*

Affect is a verb meaning to influence, act upon, change, modify or alter. If you can substitute the words in parentheses below and preserve the desired meaning of the sentence, then the word *affect* or *affects* is probably appropriate.

▶ **Example:** The presence of velopharyngeal incompetence *affects* (*influences, acts upon, changes, modifies, alters*) the child's performance on the *Iowa Pressure Articulation Test* (IPAT).

Affect can also be used as a noun depicting the inward feeling or disposition.

▶ **Example:** Her affect appeared quiet and melancholy.

Table 2.4
Positive Terminology for Describing Behavior

Negative	Positive
laziness	can perform better when motivated
troublemaker	disturbs the class
uncooperative	needs to learn to work with others
cheats	depends on others' work
stupid	needs help
below average	is performing at own level
dirty	poor self-care habits
uninterested	complacent
must	should
stubborn	strong-willed
insolent	outspoken
liar	tends to stretch the truth
wastes time	needs to make better use of time
sloppy	needs to do neater work
failed	did not meet the requirements
nasty	has difficulty getting along with others
time and again	usually
poor work	work below usual standards
clumsy	awkward motor movements
profane	uses unacceptable language
selfish	needs to share more with others
rude	inconsiderate of feelings of others
bashful	shy; reserved
showoff	tries to get attention

Note. From *School Programs in Speech–Language: Organization and Management*, by E. Neidecker and J. Blosser, 1993, Needham Heights, MA: Allyn & Bacon. Copyright 1993 by Allyn & Bacon. Reprinted with permission.

Effect is a verb meaning to cause, make, achieve, execute, or bring about. If you can substitute the words in parentheses below and preserve the desired meaning of the sentence, then the word *effect* or *effects* is probably appropriate.

▶ **Example:** The use of easy onset phonation *effects* (*causes, makes, achieves, executes, brings about*) a positive change in phonatory quality.

The word *effect* can also be used as a noun conveying the outcome, result, or conclusion. If you can substitute the words in parentheses below and preserve the desired meaning of the sentence, then the word *effect* is probably appropriate.

▶ **Example:** A positive *effect* (*outcome, result, conclusion*) of treatment is improved social skills.

For practice using these terms, complete the exercises on Worksheet 2.

Amount and Number

Amount is a noun that refers to quantity, sum, whole, mass, or total.

▶ **Example:** The *amount* and extent of vagus nerve involvement described in the medical report explain the primary etiology for the client's voice disorder.

Number is a noun that refers to units that can be counted.

▶ **Example:** The *number* of correct responses increases when the words are modeled by the examiner.

The word *number* can also be used as a verb meaning enumerate, list, count, tally, compute, figure, or calculate.

▶ **Example:** The client will *number* the correct responses listed in his notebook and graph the totals at the end of each week.

For practice using these terms, complete Worksheet 3.

Anxious and Eager

Anxious refers to a state of distress, concern, apprehension, nervousness, or fear.

▶ **Example:** Ms. Hermosillo seems *anxious* about her child's readiness for first grade.

Eager is used to express desire, zeal, and enthusiasm.

▶ **Example:** The child is *eager* to complete all activities.

Worksheet 4 provides practice using these terms.

Can and May

Can implies the ability to do something.

▶ **Example:** Mrs. Moreno *can* effectively swallow thickened liquids.

May implies permission or degree of probability.

▶ **Example:** The client's swallowing difficulties *may* be related to the following factors.

For practice using these terms, complete Worksheet 5.

(*text continues on p. 18*)

Worksheet 1

Preferred Terminology

After reviewing the sample, rewrite the following sentences using preferred terminology.

1. Sean, a victim of Mongolism and mental retardation, is severely delayed in speech and language development.

   Rewrite: <u>Sean has Down syndrome accompanied by mental retardation and a severe delay in speech and language development.</u>

2. Angelina's articulation is typical of articulation errors found in "deafy" speech.

   _____

   _____

3. Valerie has arthritis and is confined to a wheelchair.

   _____

   _____

4. Defective at birth, Don is an epileptic and an invalid.

   _____

   _____

5. Kathryn's seizure disorder has rendered her an academic failure.

   _____

   _____

6. Fred, though able-bodied, is deaf and blind.

   _____

   _____

7. Harvey is rude, insolent, and uncooperative.

   _____

   _____

8. Gay used profane language as she failed the tests administered.

   _____

   _____

(continues)

Worksheet 1 *(Continued)*

9. Mary's laziness contributes to her poor work in the academic setting.

_____

_____

10. Ricardo appeared uninterested and somewhat bashful during the evaluation.

_____

_____

11. Bryan is a troublemaker and cheats in class.

_____

_____

12. Grace was defective at birth with a cleft palate, has been spoiled and tends to be selfish and rude.

_____

_____

13. Don is clumsy, does sloppy work, uses profanity in class, and is a really big showoff.

_____

_____

14. Time and again, Kay fails examinations administered in class.

_____

_____

15. Insolent and stubborn, Bobby Joe refuses to cooperate in the clinical setting.

_____

_____

Compare your revisions with those of others. Notice how many different ways one might write these sentences, using appropriate terminology and positive behavioral descriptions.

Table 2.5

ICD Classifications that Pertain to Speech–Language Pathology and Audiology

290.0	Senile Dementia (Uncomplicated)		388.31	Subjective Tinnitus
290.1	Presenile Dementia (Brain Syndrome)		388.32	Objective Tinnitus
290.10	Presenile Dementia (Uncomplicated)		388.40	Abnormal Auditory Perception; Unspecified
299	Infantile Autism		388.41	Diplacusis
307.0	Stuttering; Stammering		388.42	Hyperacusis
307.3	Stereotyped Repetitive Movements (body rocking; head banging)		388.43	Impairment of Auditory Discrimination
			388.44	Recruitment
307.9	Other Unspecified Special Symptoms or Syndromes (including lalling, lisping)		388.5	Impairment Acoustic Nerve
			389.00	Conductive Hearing Loss, Unspecified
309.83	Elective Mutism (with no adjustment reaction)		389.01	Conductive Hearing Loss, External Ear
313.23	Elective Mutism (adjustment reaction with withdrawal)		389.02	Conductive Hearing Loss, Tympanic Membrane
314.00	Attention Deficit Disorder; no hyperactivity (inattentive)		389.03	Conductive Hearing Loss, Middle Ear
			389.04	Conductive Hearing Loss, Inner Ear
314.01	Attention Deficit Disorder; with hyperactivity		389.08	Conductive Hearing Loss, Combined Types
315	Specific Delays in Development		389.1	Sensorineural Hearing Loss
315.00	Specific Reading Disorder; Unspecified		389.2	Mixed Conductive and Sensorineural Hearing Loss
315.01	Alexia		389.7	Deaf; nonspeaking
315.02	Developmental Dyslexia		478.30	Paralysis of Vocal Cords or Larynx; Unspecified
315.1	Specific Arithmetical Disorder (acalculia)		478.31	Unilateral Paralysis; Partial
315.2	Other Specific Learning Difficulties		478.32	Unilateral Paralysis; Complete
315.3	Developmental Speech or Language Disorder		478.33	Bilateral Paralysis; Partial
315.31	Developmental Language Disorder; Developmental Aphasia; Word Deafness		478.34	Bilateral Paralysis; Complete
			478.4	Polyps of Vocal Cords or Larynx
315.39	Other (Developmental Articulation Disorder; Dyslalia)		478.5	Other Diseases of Vocal Cords
315.4	Coordination Disorder (Dyspraxia Syndrome)		478.6	Edema of Larynx
315.5	Mixed Development Disorder		478.74	Stenosis of Larynx
315.8	Other Specified Delays in Development		478.75	Laryngeal Spasm
315.9	Unspecified Delay in Development		530.81	Esophageal Reflux
317	Mild Mental Retardation		749.0	Cleft Palate; Unspecified
318	Moderate Mental Retardation		749.01	Cleft Palate; Unilateral Complete
318.1	Severe Mental Retardation		749.02	Cleft Palate: Unilateral Incomplete
319	Unspecified Mental Retardation		749.03	Cleft Palate; Bilateral Complete
388	Degenerative and Vascular Disorders of the Ear		749.04	Cleft Palate; Bilateral Incomplete
388.01	Presbycusis		749.10	Cleft Lip; Unspecified
388.02	Transient Ischemic Deafness		749.11	Cleft Lip; Unilateral Complete
388.1	Noise Affects on Inner Ear; Unspecified		749.12	Cleft Lip; Unilateral Incomplete
388.11	Acoustic Trauma (explosive)		749.13	Cleft Lip; Bilateral Complete
388.12	Noise Induced Hearing Loss		749.14	Cleft Lip; Bilateral Incomplete
388.2	Sudden Hearing Loss; Unspecified			
388.30	Tinnitus; Unspecified			

(continues)

Table 2.5 (*Continued*)

749.20	Cleft Lip and Palate; Unspecified	780.4	Dizziness and Giddiness
749.21	Cleft Lip and Palate; Unilateral Complete	780.5	Sleep Disturbances
749.22	Cleft Lip and Palate; Unilateral Incomplete	781	Symptoms Involving Nervous and Musculoskeletal Systems
749.23	Cleft Lip and Palate; Bilateral Complete	781.0	Abnormal Involuntary Movements
749.24	Cleft Lip and Palate; Bilateral Incomplete	781.1	Disturbances of Sensation of Smell and Taste
749.25	Other Combinations	781.2	Abnormality of Gait
750.0	Ankyloglossia	781.3	Lack of Coordination
750.10	Anomaly of Tongue; Unspecified	783.3	Feeding Problems (Elderly/Infants)
750.11	Aglossia	783.4	Failure to Thrive
750.12	Congenital Adhesions of Tongue	784.0	Headache
750.13	Fissure of Tongue	784.1	Throat Pain
750.15	Macroglossia	784.2	Swelling, Mass or Lump in Head/Neck
750.16	Microglossia	784.3	Aphasia (excludes developmental aphasia)
779.3	Feeding Disturbance (In Newborn)	784.4	Voice Disturbances; Unspecified
780.00	Alteration of Consciousness	784.41	Aphonia
780.01	Coma	784.5	Other Speech Disturbance (Dysarthria, Dysphasia; Slurred Speech)
780.02	Transient Alteration of Awareness		
780.03	Persistent Vegetative State	784.6	Other Symbolic Dysfunction; Unspecified
780.09	Other (drowsiness, semicoma, unconsciousness, somnolence (sleepiness), stupor)	784.61	Alexia and Dyslexia
		784.69	Other (Acalculia, Agnosia, Agraphia, Apraxia)
780.1	Hallucinations	786	Dyspnea and Respiratory Abnormalities
780.2	Syncope and Collapse (blackout, fainting, presyncope)	786.1	Congenital Laryngeal Stridor
780.3	Convulsions	787.2	Dysphagia

Note. From *International Classification of Diseases–Ninth Edition*, by U.S. Department of Health and Human Services, 1994, Washington, DC: Public Health Services and Health Care Financing Administration.

Table 2.6
Guidelines for Composing Readable Reports

1. Use simple vocabulary and natural sentence structure. Limit sentence length to 18 words or less and paragraph length to 125 words or less.

2. Delete the words *that, by, which, who,* and *whom,* then reconstruct the sentence without them.

3. Choose short words over long ones.

4. Write in the active voice when possible.

5. Remove qualifying adjectives such as *very, quite, much, rather, somewhat,* and *approximately.*

6. Nouns ending in *ion* should be changed to verbs. For example, "Her verbalizations were short" would be changed to, "She verbalized in short utterances."

7. Vary the length and type of sentences.

8. Make revisions, then read the report aloud while judging whether the report would make sense to others having only the report in front of them.

9. Revise further with the objectives of making the complex more simple and the unfamiliar more familiar.

Note. From "Editor's Notebook: Texas Talk," by R. Reece, 1982, *Minnesota Medicine, 65*(12). Copyright 1982 by Minnesota Medicine. Reprinted with permission.

Further and *Farther*

Further is used with caution. *Further* relates to additional or extra time.

▶ **Example:** Before *further* work is done on this objective, additional testing is needed.

Usually a sentence reads better if the word *more* is substituted for the word *further*.

▶ **Example:** Before *more* work is done on this objective, additional testing is needed.

The word *furthermore* is often used for transition, meaning *in addition*.

▶ **Example:** *Furthermore*, if additional testing reveals that the child's language function is commensurate with his developmental age, then treatment should be discontinued.

Farther refers to distance.

▶ **Example:** Without assistance, Joey refused to walk farther today than he walked last week.

i.e. and *e.g.*

The abbreviation *i.e.* stands for *id est*, which means "that is."

▶ **Example:** Her speech intelligibility, *i.e.*, her ability to be understood by unfamiliar listeners, is poor.

The abbreviation *e.g.* stands for *exempli gratia*, which means "for example."

▶ **Example:** Carolyn occasionally repeats syllables (*e.g.*, "dada").

Exercise

Select the appropriate abbreviations:

1. Doug substituted [w] for [l] (*i.e./e.g.*, "wamp" for "lamp").
2. Her diadochokinetic rates (*i.e./e.g.*, her ability to articulate timed sequenced syllables) are slow and imprecise in specificity and range of lingual movements.

(**Answers:** 1. e.g.; 2. i.e.)

Immediately, Presently, and *Currently*

Immediately means instantly, right now, without delay, or at once.

▶ **Example:** Based on Crista's tympanogram and her report of pain in the right ear, she should see an otologist *immediately*.

Presently means soon, shortly, or before long. The reference is to the near future.

▶ **Example:** Ms. Walker reports that she should (*presently*) *soon* receive an answer from her insurance carrier regarding coverage for speech and language services. The word *soon* is more direct and sounds less dated than the word *presently*. However, *presently* often is used incorrectly to replace the word *currently*.

Currently refers to the prevailing condition or time. Often the sentence reads just as well when the word *currently* is omitted altogether.

▶ **Example:** Kelley is (*currently*) teaching the third grade at Copeland Elementary School.

Exercise

Select the appropriate word in the following sentences:

1. José is (*immediately/presently/soon/currently*) practicing production of [r] in specific phonetic contexts identified by *Deep Test of Articulation* as those he can produce correctly.
2. Mary Lou will (*immediately/presently/soon/currently*) be given an appointment to see a counselor at the Child Development Center.
3. Based on observed seizurelike behavior, it is recommended that Mark see a neurologist (*immediately/presently/soon/currently*).

(**Answers:** 1. currently; 2. soon; 3. immediately)

Confused Relationships

In addition to incorrect word choice, accuracy may be sacrificed by the use of confused relationships that cause confusion in logic.

▶ **Example:** Because she is in the first grade, Julia's articulation should be reevaluated in the fall.

One might rewrite this so that a logical basis is provided for the retesting.

▶ **Example:** Julia's articulation errors seem to be developmental. When she enters second grade next year, her articulation should be reassessed to monitor its development.

Clarity of written information may be compromised by repetitious or redundant usage of words, phrases, and ideas.

Word Repetition

Reported and *stated* are often repeated throughout the history section in an attempt to clearly identify the provider of specific

(text continues on p. 23)

Worksheet 2

Use of *Affect* and *Effect*

Mark a plus (+) if the sentence is correct, a minus (−) if it is incorrect.

_____ Johnny's attitude effects his performance.

_____ The use of visual cues effects increased stimulability in correct articulator placement for production of lingua-alveolar consonants.

_____ The parents feel that Mildred's friends negatively affect her self-image as a speaker.

_____ Phyllis reports her mother's suggestions for improving fluency had a beneficial affect.

_____ The positive affects of reading to preschool-aged children on their speech and language development are documented by research.

(**Answers:** −, −, +, +, −)

Choose the correct form of *affect* or *effect* in these sentences.

1. Myrna's regular practice sessions using reduced rate and an easy relaxed approach (affects/effects) improved fluency in conversational speech.

2. John's (affect/effect) during the fluency-enhancing exercise was flat and emotionless.

3. Feared speaking situations negatively (affect/effect) John's fluency.

4. Phonological treatment generally has a positive (affect/effect) on speech intelligibility.

5. A change in Jacob's home environment appeared to have a positive (affect/effect).

6. Joe Bubba's weak performance on the *Test of Language Development–Primary: Third Edition* appeared to be (affected/effected) by short attention and behavioral difficulties.

7. Gary's motivation to increase his fluency skills should have a positive (affect/effect) on the prognosis for his speech improvement.

8. (Affected/Effected) by the presence of her mother, Elsie was frequently distracted while taking the *Test of Language Development–Primary: Third Edition.*

9. Tom's improved fluency appears to be (affected/effected) primarily by his use of rate control and voluntary stuttering.

10. Loud sound (affects/effects) in movie theaters cause Marjorie to cry and cover her ears.

(**Answers:** 1. effects; 2. affect; 3. affect; 4. effect; 5. effect; 6. affected; 7. effect; 8. Affected; 9. effected; 10. effects)

Worksheet 3

Use of *Amount* and *Number*

Mark a plus (+) if the sentence is correct, a minus (−) if it is incorrect.

_____ The amount of grammatical errors did not change with increased length and complexity of utterance.

_____ The number of opportunities for deletion of stridency was determined from the speech sample and compared with the actual number of times the phonological rule was used.

_____ The amount of speech improvement varied according to the child's general health.

_____ The number of Chad's dysfluencies per 100 words varied from three to eight words, depending on the speaking situation.

_____ Vicki's parents are concerned about the amount of time it will take to improve her speech intelligibility.

(**Answers:** − , + , + , + , +)

Fill in the blank with the correct word (*amount* or *number*).

1. The _____ of responses varied with the type of activity.

2. Carmen enjoyed computing and graphing the _____ of her correct responses following treatment each day.

3. Her correct responses increased in _____ when she began receiving individual treatment sessions.

4. The _____ of treatment time spent on vocabulary drills each day averaged 20 minutes.

5. She needs to be referred for a complete audiological examination to determine the _____ of hearing loss in her left ear.

6. Joe's high _____ of vocal abuses during playground activities appears related to his difficulty in getting along with peers.

7. During a five-minute conversation, Dolly was dysfluent on five words, an/a _____ felt to be within general normal limits.

8. The _____ of sessions scheduled weekly during the spring term will depend upon availability of public transportation for adults with physical disabilities.

9. The _____ of treatment needed to improve a client's performance is based upon a _____ of factors.

10. The client will _____ his correct responses using a hand counter.

(**Answers:** 1. number; 2. number; 3. amount; 4. amount; 5. amount; 6. number; 7. number; 8. number; 9. amount, number; 10. number)

Worksheet 4

Use of *Anxious* and *Eager*

Select *anxious* or *eager* as the appropriate word to complete each of these sentences.

1. Ms. Goldman was _____ to have her child enrolled in speech and language treatment.

2. Ms. Bernstein guardedly and _____ly reported the details of her son's previous history of emotional problems.

3. Mr. Rodriguez indicated that he is _____ to begin a treatment program designed to help him cope with his stuttering.

4. Carole _____ly completed the activities and resisted leaving the room when the session was over.

5. Although she entered the clinical setting _____ly, Sophia appeared to relax and enjoy the fluency-enhancing activities as she developed confidence.

6. Ginger's mother appeared _____ when the potential benefits of enrolling the child in preschool were presented.

7. At the end of the session, Mr. Reagan appeared tired and nervous. He _____ly waited for his wife to pick him up.

8. Carlos was not _____ to complete any of the formal tests administered.

9. Despite her lack of attention and refusal to complete most activities presented, Olivia _____ly completed all of the receptive items needed to reach a ceiling score on the *Preschool Language Scale*.

10. Ms. Jackson reported that Andrew's eye–hand coordination is regressing. She is _____ to enroll him in physical therapy.

11. Mr. Hymel responds best to treatment during early afternoon sessions. During morning sessions he tends to be impatient and _____ about a variety of factors that he finds worrisome.

12. Grace appears _____ to enroll in treatment but seems _____ about the possibility of being assigned a male clinician.

13. The child's grandmother is _____ about our recommendation for the child's velopharyngeal function to be assessed by a craniofacial team. She is _____ly attempting to convince the child's parents to ignore the recommendation and seek a second opinion.

14. It appears that Janie's prognosis for improvement with treatment is good based on her cooperation in the clinical setting and Ms. Littlebear's expressed _____ness to be actively involved in the treatment process.

15. Mr. Nickel was _____ to finish the session early.

(**Answers:** 1. eager; 2. anxiously; 3. eager; 4. eagerly; 5. anxiously; 6. eager; 7. anxiously; 8. eager; 9. anxiously; 10. eager; 11. anxious; 12. eager, anxious; 13. anxious, eagerly; 14. eagerness; 15. eager.)

Worksheet 5

Use of *Can* and *May*

Fill in the blank with the appropriate word (*can* or *may*).

1. The child's errored production of the [r] phoneme _____ be related to a lack of precision and specificity of lingual movement.

2. The child _____ count to 10 and recite the alphabet, short poems, and rhymes.

3. Jackie's hypernasal resonance _____ be attributed to the presence of an unoperated velar cleft palate.

4. Elsa has a mild to moderate delay in the acquisition of speech and language, which _____ be related to the presence of a moderate bilateral mixed hearing loss.

5. Betty _____ name selected common objects with 80% accuracy.

6. Murphy _____ eat solid foods and drink liquids without aspirating.

7. Ada _____ attend to a task for two to three minutes.

8. Ms. Peña reported that John _____ dress himself.

9. Ms. Wieznewsky stated that she thinks Alvin's unintelligible speech and limited vocabulary _____ be related to his previously frequent episodes of otitis media.

10 Cel's phonatory hoarseness _____ be related to episodes of coughing that accompany her asthmatic condition.

11. Based upon observation of Jimmy's behavior during the evaluation, it was concluded that he _____ benefit from treatment provided that the family is willing to participate in an accompanying structured home program.

12. Based upon observation during the initial speech and language evaluation, it was determined that Mrs. Hollingsworth _____ follow simple instructions.

13. Based on this assessment, Elwood _____ not safely swallow liquids while using compensatory swallowing strategies.

14. Jack _____ retrieve single words if given initial sound cues.

15. Severely involved clients _____ generally benefit from an expanded treatment program coordinated between school and university clinicians.

(**Answers:** 1. may; 2. can; 3. may; 4. may; 5. can; 6. can; 7. can; 8. can; 9. may; 10. may; 11. may; 12. can; 13. can; 14. can; 15. can)

information. Other words that can be used to reduce overuse of these words include *indicated, remarked, observed, asserted, said, described, revealed, related, disclosed, added,* and *noted.*

Adequate and *adequately* and *reported* and *reportedly* are often repeated in the examination findings section of a report. Other options might include the words *sufficient* or *sufficiently; enough; competent* or *competently; appropriate* or *appropriately; acceptable* or *acceptably; satisfactory* or *satisfactorily; ample; effectual* or *effectually.*

For practice, review a diagnostic report (either from your files or in the samples provided in this book) and note the words that are used to convey *adequate* performance in the examination and the *report* of information in the history. List them, then list alternative word choices.

Redundancy and Wordiness

Following are examples of redundancy (and thus wordiness) in phrasing and ideas. Identify a word (either a new word or one of the words included in the wordy phrase) that could substitute for each phrase. Worksheet 6 provides practice in editing wordy phrases.

Wordy Phrase	Revision
may possibly	may
might possibly	might
small in size	small
normal and no complications	normal
prior or previous history	prior history
absolutely essential	essential
future plans	plans
various different	different
spell out in detail	describe
qualified expert	expert
advanced planning	preparation
each and every	each; every
at this point in time	currently
certainly inappropriate	inappropriate
totally involved	involved
successfully produced	produced
the true fact	the fact
several different types	several types; different types
as of yet	(omit entirely)
far and above	exceed; surpass

One simple rule facilitates clarity: When a single word will effectively convey the intended meaning, use it. Of course there are exceptions. The intent of the clinician and the language in common professional use must also be considered.

Table 2.7 provides examples of simple words that can be substituted for more complex ones.

Transition

Transitional phrases facilitate the smooth flow of sentences and paragraphs. There is a tendency to overuse certain transitional phrases and connectives. Table 2.8 provides some alternatives for transitions that lend variety and decrease repetition.

Of course, sometimes simple, overused words are replaced with more complex or longer words. However, in the interest of creating a readable report, it is sometimes advisable to sacrifice simplicity for smooth transition. Review a diagnostic report and note where transitional phrases and words could be placed for variety and ease of reading.

Use of Pronouns

If the writer has mentioned more than one person before using a pronoun to refer to one of them, confusion is certain to result. Sometimes pronouns are placed too far from the noun they relate to, causing the pronoun to drift. In any case, the noun should be restated.

In the following example, clarity suffers because of pronoun misuse and wordiness.

▶ **History:** Ms. Garcia described her pregnancy with Dawn as being normal with no complicating factors. However, one week following her birth, Ms. Garcia had occasion to be hospitalized due to a uterine infection. She was cared for by her father during this particular time.

The example might be rewritten as follows:

▶ **History:** Ms. Garcia's pregnancy with Dawn was unremarkable. One week following her birth, Dawn was cared for by her father while Ms. Garcia was hospitalized for a uterine infection.

During editing, the writer might decide that Dawn's caretaker during her mother's hospitalization was not relevant and delete reference to it.

There is disagreement about the use of personal pronouns in report writing. W. O. Haynes and Pindzola (1998) believe that personal pronouns should be avoided; in other words that "it is preferable to keep the 'I' out of it" because an impersonal writing style minimizes "the writer's verbal idiosyncrasies" and also tends to facilitate objectivity (p. 411). They recommend that reference be made to the "examiner" or the "clinician" to maintain a more impersonal style. Knepflar (1976), on the other hand, maintains that personal pronouns should be used when they are the natural way to make a clear statement, and that to avoid using personal pronouns can give the impression

Worksheet 6

Editing Wordy Phrases

Choose from the following list a word to replace each wordy phrase listed below.

about	can	felt	later	possibly
although	cannot	few	many	repeatedly
analyzes	consider	fewer	much	to
apparently	describes	frequently	now	was
because	evidently	if	obviously	when
believes	feels	in	often	while
by				

Wordy Phrase	Reader's Response	Wordy Phrase	Reader's Response
1. the fact that	_____	17. considerable number of	_____
2. at the present time	_____	18. during the time that	_____
3. at this point in time	_____	19. it may be said that	_____
4. in view of the fact that	_____	20. over and over	_____
5. small numbers of	_____	21. despite the fact that	_____
6. at some future time	_____	22. presents an analysis of	_____
7. within the area of	_____	23. it is often the case that	_____
8. relative to	_____	24. by means of	_____
9. gives a description of	_____	25. in the event that	_____
10. considerable amount of	_____	26. has the ability to	_____
11. it is apparent that	_____	27. in order to	_____
12. is unable to	_____	28. for the reason that	_____
13. take into consideration	_____	29. be of the opinion that	_____
14. owing to the fact that	_____	30. it would appear that	_____
15. decrease in the number of	_____	31. had occasion to be	_____
16. as of now	_____		

(**Suggested Responses:** 1. because; 2. now; 3. now; 4. apparently; 5. few; 6. later; 7. in; 8. about; 9. describes; 10. much; 11. obviously, apparently; 12. cannot; 13. consider; 14. because; 15. fewer; 16. now; 17. many; 18. while; 19. possibly; 20. frequently, repeatedly; 21. although; 22. analyzes; 23. often, frequently; 24. by; 25. if; 26. can; 27. to; 28. because; 29. believes, feels; 30. apparently; 31. was)

Table 2.7

Word Pairs: Simple and Complex

Simple	Complex
advanced	sophisticated, progressive
after	following, beyond
answer	reply, respond
begin or start	commence, initiate, originate
do	accomplish, achieve, execute, perform, effect, complete
end	terminate, finish, complete, conclude, discontinue
enough	sufficient, plenty, adequate, ample, abundant
expect	anticipate, await, foresee, envision, require, assume
find	locate, detect, discover, recover, retrieve, determine
get	acquire, obtain, secure, procure
happen or occur	transpire, ensue, take place
help	assist, serve, facilitate, improve
hopeful	optimistic, encouraging, promising
keep	retain, reserve, maintain
know	realize, comprehend, discern, understand, perceive
later	subsequently, afterward, consequently, following
live	reside, dwell
met	encountered
more	greater
much	substantial, abundant, ample, considerable
new	sophisticated, innovative, inventive, current
on	upon
say	remark, state, articulate, speak, express, relate, declare
seem	appear
send	transmit, direct, refer, route, relay
show	demonstrate, exhibit, reveal, display, perform, present
so	thus
try	endeavor, attempt, undertake, venture
use	operate, manipulate, utilize, employ, expend, consume

that the writer is not willing to take responsibility. Somewhere between these views, Peterson and Marquardt (1994) indicated that an impersonal and relatively formal tone should be maintained in reporting, although personal pronouns should be used when they are the most appropriate way to make a clear statement.

Avoiding personal pronouns promotes use of the passive style of sentence construction. Some believe that active sentence construction should be used whenever possible, while passive forms should be avoided (APA, 1994; Meitus, 1983). Thus, the writer must decide whether to use personal pronouns in report writing. The purpose and recipients of the report, along with the usual style preferred by the agency, will influence the writer's decision. Most important, the writer should be consistent in the use of personal pronouns and active or passive voice within sections of a single report.

Style: Common Errors

Style is improved by consistency in voice and tense and in spelling, punctuation, sentence structure, and expression of numbers. Use of folksy or cute phrasing quickly reduces the level of professionalism conveyed by the report. Following are exercises to provide the clinician with practice in editing reports to improve style.

Consistency in Voice and Tense

Active voice is more direct and livelier to read. Passive voice is justified if the actor is less important than what is acted upon. Consistent use of the past tense usually is appropriate in the history section of a report. However, consistent use of the present tense is appropriate when describing the performance at the time of the assessment along with the impressions and recommendations.

▶ **History example:** It is reported by Ms. Espinoza that Albert's speech and language development is slower than that of his older brother.

▶ **Edited version:** Ms. Espinoza reported that Albert's speech and language development was slower than that of his older brother.

▶ **Examination example:** Debra's receptive language abilities were revealed by her performance at the 3-year, 6-month level on the *OWLS Listening Comprehension Scale*.

▶ **Edited version:** Debra's performance on the *OWLS Listening Comprehension Scale* places her at the 3½ year level in receptive language.

▶ **Impressions example:** Marcie was diagnosed as being a severe stutterer characterized by struggle behaviors, part-word repetitions, and whole-word repetitions. I think her prognosis for improvement with treatment is good because she has a positive attitude and can modify her speech.

Table 2.8
Transitional Words and Phrases for Variety

Connectives Between Paragraphs

accordingly	consequently	in fact	similarly
also	conversely	likewise	such
another	finally	moreover	then
as a result	for example	nevertheless	therefore
at last	for instance	on the other hand	thus
at this time	furthermore	otherwise	too

Transitions Reflecting Logical Conclusion

accordingly	consequently	therefore
as a result	hence	thus

Words and Phrases for Contrast or Objection

but	on the contrary	on the other hand
however	conversely	whereas

Phrases Noting Concession

to be certain	given that	being assured
granted that	no doubt	

Phrases for Introducing an Illustration

as an example	for example	in particular
as an illustration	for instance	

Phrases Introducing Paraphrase or Summary

in other words	in summary	in effect	to conclude
in short	in brief	that is	

Frequently Used Transitional Expressions

hence	nevertheless	since	therefore
however	nonetheless	though	thus

Common Adverbs Reflecting Conjunctions

and	also, furthermore, in addition, incidentally, in turn, moreover, once again, similarly, then, too
but	actually, although, anyhow, anyway, at any rate, at the same time, by contrast, by the same token, conversely, either, however, in any case, in any event, in reality, instead, neither, nevertheless, nonetheless, of course, on the contrary, on the other hand, to be sure
or	conversely, either, neither, in reverse, on the other hand
so	accordingly, as a result, consequently, hence, then, therefore, thus
for	above all, after all, additionally, besides, as a matter of fact, at least, certainly, first of all, for one thing, in brief, in fact, in short, in the first place, indeed, likewise, secondly

▶ **Edited version:** Marcie presents a severe stuttering disorder characterized by struggle behaviors and part- and whole-word repetitions. Prognosis for improvement with treatment appears good based on her positive attitude and ability to modify her speech with instruction.

▶ **Recommendations example:** I recommend that Ms. Pisell's larynx be evaluated by an otolaryngologist before she begins vocal health instruction.

▶ **Edited version:** Ms. Pisell should be seen by an otolaryngologist for a laryngeal examination. Based on the results of that evaluation, she may be a good candidate for vocal health instruction.

Elimination of Folksy or Colloquial Phrasing

The writer should weigh carefully whether to use the words *rather, very, little, pretty,* and *some.* Usually they can be deleted. Phrases like *bored to death, pretty cooperative, very tired, way past, not too long ago, pretty well, rather anxious, a little feverish,* and *some candy* (as reinforcers) are examples of folksy or colloquial phrases that have been included in diagnostic reports. Every writer must maintain vigilance in editing such phrases from reports and other professional correspondence.

Consistency in Spelling

Some words have two accepted spellings (e.g., *cuing* or *cueing*). One selected spelling must be used consistently throughout the report.

Proofreading carefully for typographical errors is essential. Some editors read the text backwards to locate misspelled words. A spell checking feature on word processing software is helpful, but one must remember that if *two* is spelled *to* or *too*, the spell check will not pick it up because all those words are spelled correctly. Reading the text aloud, proofreading by peers or supervisors dedicated to protecting confidentiality, and setting the report aside for 24 hours and then rereading it are other strategies some find helpful in locating errors.

Some adjectives may be used differently depending on *–ic* or *–ical* endings. The American Medical Association Press (Fishbein, 1950) has adopted a list of preferred endings. See Table 2.9 for a list of adjectives that appear most often in the reports of speech–language pathologists and audiologists.

Consistency with Numbers

Numbers one through nine should be written out as words unless the number is a unit of measure, such as a time, date, age, page number, percentage, unit of money, test score, or score on a scale. Numbers 10 and above should be expressed as figures. If a number lower than 10 appears in the same sentence for comparison with a number 10 or above, then it is expressed as a figure. The following are sentences that need editing for number use:

▶ **Example:** Judy walked at nine months, said her first word at eighteen months, and appropriately used two-word phrases at 2 years.

▶ **Edited version:** Judy walked at 9 months, said her first word at 18 months, and appropriately used two-word phrases at 2 years. (The edited version shows consistent use of figures to designate age.)

▶ **Example:** On the *Assessment of Phonological Processes–Revised,* Sergio omitted syllables five percent of the possible occurrences, reduced consonant sequences 55 percent of the possible occurrences, omitted prevocalic consonant singletons five percent of the possible occurrences, produced no stridents or liquid [l] and [r] phonemes, and produced velar obstruents fifty-nine percent of the possible occurrences and glides thirty percent of the possible occurrences.

▶ **Edited version:** Sergio's responses to the *Assessment of Phonological Processes–Revised* provides a phonological analysis of his production of 50 selected words. Of the possible number of occurrences on the assessment, Sergio's percentage of usage of the phonological processes is as follows: Omission of Syllables (5%); Reduction of Consonant Sequences (55%); Omission of Prevocalic Consonant Singletons (5%); Production of Velar Obstruents (59%); and Production of Glides (30%). Sergio produced no strident or liquid [l] or [r] patterns. (All percentages are in figures.)

Consistency in Punctuation

Writers often find quotations and phrases within parentheses difficult to punctuate. Confusion usually lies in placement of punctuation inside or outside quotation marks or parentheses. Commas and periods are placed inside quotation marks unless a parenthetical reference is included. Parentheses enclose matter apart from the main thought.

▶ **Example without parentheses:** Jasper's speech is characterized by the use of structurally incomplete utterances that convey complete thoughts. Following is a short segment of the sample: "Boy go no bye bye." "We see doggie." "I no see bear." "We like nice doggie."

Table 2.9

Preferred Adjectives with –*ic* and –*ical* Endings

The parallel adjective forms created by the endings –*ic* and –*ical* may be used interchangeably. However, –*ic* may be used to denote a closer relationship with the root word, and –*ical* may denote a more general theory or system.

–*ic* = of, pertaining to, or belonging to; connected with; dealing with

–*ical* = theory; system; disorder; skills

Adjective	Definition	Example
acoustic	pertaining to perception	acoustic phonetics
acoustical	serving to aid hearing	acoustical aid
anatomic	relating to anatomy	anatomic structures
anatomical	structural theory	anatomical system
audiologic	connected with hearing	audiologic habilitation
audiological	related to study of hearing	audiological evaluation
biologic	pertaining to study of life	biologic features
biological	used in applied biology	biological supplies
chronologic	pertaining to chronology	chronologic events
chronological	events in order of time	chronological age
diacritic	denoting phonetic difference	diacritic mark
diacritical	system to distinguish form/sound	diacritical transcription of letters/phonemes
embryologic	dealing with study of embryo	embryologic feature
embryological	theory related to embryology	embryological research
grammatic	pertaining to grammar	grammatic closure
grammatical	grammar system/theory	grammatical analysis
hierarchic	pertaining to series	hierarchic order
hierarchical	system for sequencing	hierarchical arrangement
laryngologic	pertaining to larynx	laryngologic structure
laryngological	laryngeal system	laryngological examination
linguistic	pertains to study of languages	linguistic component
linguistical	study of language theory	linguistical analysis
morphologic	pertains to morphology	morphologic construction
morphological	component pertaining to morphological skills	formulation of words
neurologic	pertains to nervous system	neurologic structure
neurological	neurological system	neurological exam
pathologic	pertains to pathology	pathologic condition
pathological	condition due to disease	pathological tissue
phonologic	pertains to sound changes	phonologic errors
phonological	theory of developmental sound	phonological theory; analysis, changes in children
physiologic	pertains to function	physiologic aspects
physiological	study of normal function	physiological abnormalities
prosodic	pertains to speech patterns	prosodic features
prosodical	theory of prosodic features	prosodical difficulties
psychologic	pertaining to psychology	psychologic considerations
psychological	theories of psychology	psychological measures
syntactic	pertaining to syntax	syntactic rule
syntactical	theory underlying rules	syntactical performance

Note. From *Medical Writing: The Technic and the Art*, by M. Fishbein, 1950, Philadelphia: McGraw-Hill. Copyright 1950 by McGraw-Hill. Reprinted with permission.

► **Example with parentheses:** Javier responded to pictures with one-word utterances (e.g., "Mommy," "baby," "kitty," and "door").

Parentheses are used to provide explanatory information. The punctuation is enclosed by the parentheses if the statement is complete. (A complete sentence is completely enclosed by parentheses.) The punctuation follows the closing parenthesis if the parenthetical word or phrase lies within the statement (including the end of the sentence). Parentheses are confusing (even for the most experienced writer).

Parallel Sentence Structure

Parallel sentence structure is often lacking in the recommendations section of a report.

► **Example of poor parallel structure:** *Recommendations*—Jeanie should be enrolled in voice treatment emphasizing the following:

1. To improve her vocal habits;

2. Provide information on the relationship between vocal habits and the condition of the vocal folds; and

3. She will become more informed on the anatomy and physiology of the vocal mechanism.

► **Edited version:** *Recommendations*—Jeanie should be enrolled in voice treatment with objectives focused on her

1. heightened awareness of the relationship between vocal fold condition and vocal habits;

2. expanded understanding of basic anatomy and physiology of the vocal mechanism; and

3. increased use of good vocal habits.

There are several other options for rewriting these recommendations using parallel structure. How would you have rewritten the section?

Writing style is individual. The task is to use precise words to convey intended meaning, avoid ambiguity, and present ideas in statements that are orderly, economical, and smooth. For some, writing is a pleasant challenge. For others who are long in ideas and short in patience, writing is tiresome, difficult, and irksome. In the clinical setting, those who dislike writing may delay report writing, placing the program out of compliance with quality-assurance criteria required for program accreditation. Programs accredited by the Professional Services Board (ASHA, 1999f) must have evidence that their policies ensure timely preparation and dissemination of reports.

Writing Reports

Planning, Preparing, and Writing the First Draft

Clinicians often procrastinate in starting a diagnostic report. Reports are easiest to write just after seeing the client. Table 2.10 outlines the steps in the diagnostic report writing process. In practice, time constraints demand skipping some of the steps, often at the expense of thoroughness in that relevant information may be omitted. For some clients omitted information may be negligible, but for others (such as clients with swallowing difficulties, progressive neurological diseases, seizure-related behaviors, etc.) omitted information could result in serious consequences. Beginning report writers should develop their skills by following all the steps in the report writing process.

It is best to begin with an outline. An outline provides a plan for the report, helps ensure clarity and consistency, breaks the report into manageable units, and helps the writer see the sequence of the report from beginning to end (Bates & Kromas, 1993; Heineman & Willis, 1988; Markman, Markman, & Waddell, 1994; Theriault, 1971). Flower (1984) cautions that an outline should be adapted in accordance with the specific purposes of each report, the setting in which it is used, and the intended readers.

Once the outline is complete, the writer begins by putting the information on paper as quickly as possible; the preliminary draft is completely written before any rewriting begins. W. O. Haynes and Pindzola (1998) suggest that when the writer meets barriers, it is best to jump over them and continue with the rest of the report. The blank spots can be completed later. Necessary revisions can also be made later. It may be helpful to make notes in the margins regarding problem areas that need to be addressed. Writers who are skillful at word processing save time during the writing and revision phases of completing a report.

It is sometimes appropriate to complete specific units of the report and assemble them later. If team members of several disciplines are contributing to the report, some of the material may need to be rearranged before the draft is completed. The integrated diagnostic report is discussed later in this chapter.

When writing a clinical report, it is essential to "emphasize new information; avoid overquantification; emphasize conclusions and recommendations rather than raw data; offer recommendations, not prescriptions; and write for a specific readership" (Flower, 1984, p. 111).

Darley (1978a) emphasizes the importance of never reporting information that is critical of other professionals or agencies, or of reporting information that has been revealed in confidence.

Quotations can be informative to readers of clinical and research reports. If it is necessary to quote a parent's or client's own words, enclose them in quotation marks. Indicate omitted words by ellipses (. . .). If words must be added, enclose

Table 2.10

Steps in Writing a Diagnostic Report

1. Determine the format for the report. (This may be dictated by the agency.)

2. Read sample reports.

3. Establish a working outline, placing pertinent information under the major headings.

4. Write, word process, or dictate the preliminary draft as quickly as possible.

5. Put away the preliminary draft of the report for a day.

6. Read the entire report aloud.

7. Check the content and organization.

8. Recheck the accuracy of scores and test interpretation.

9. Correct and improve the style.

10. Correct the edited report.

11. Ask for suggestions from carefully selected reviewers who protect client confidentiality.

12. Make any changes to the report based on suggestions by reviewers with strong writing and editing skills.

13. Proofread the report carefully. Recheck spelling, punctuation, and grammar.

14. Read the report aloud once more to check for unity.

15. Make final corrections, print and sign the report.

Note. Adapted from Bates and Kromas (1993); Flower (1984); W. O. Haynes and Pindzola (1998); Markman, Markman, and Waddell (1994); Pannbacker (1975); and Theriault (1971).

them in brackets ([ ]). Markman et al. (1994) advise the writer to make certain that quoted information reads like an integral part of the report.

Several technical points warrant discussion. The preliminary draft should be saved using word processing software. The draft should be double- or triple-spaced. Pages should be numbered, and margins spaced so there is room for notations.

Revising and Refining

According to Theriault (1971), "revision . . . involves three separate and distinct operations: (1) checking the content and organization; (2) correcting and improving the style; and (3) correcting and improving the format" (p. 83). Consider these points from the reader's point of view. It may be appropriate to complete the draft, set it aside, and later begin the revision process by reading through the entire report aloud. This allows the writer to further consider the content of the report with objectivity and an eye for error.

Markman et al. (1994) suggest checking to ensure that (a) the rules for good sentence structure and style have been followed; (b) smooth transitions have been made; (c) the finished report seems logical; and (d) repetition of facts or details has been avoided. The clinician also should recheck the accuracy of all test scores and test interpretations.

Selecting the appropriate words is important. Choose specific words and consider the literacy levels of the intended readers. Technical terminology may need to be defined. Clinicians must use language commensurate with their professional competence and experience. The dictionary and thesaurus should be consulted as necessary. The following publications may also be of value: *Terminology of Communication Disorders* (Nicolosi, Harryman, & Kresheck, 1996), *Sisson's Word and Expression Locater* (Sisson, 1994), *Words Into Type* (Skillin & Gay, 1974), and *Words Fail Me* (O'Conner, 1999).

Peer review is helpful in making final revisions. Reviewers should be chosen wisely. Good reviewers protect client confidentiality, are good writers, and provide positive critical review. Editing by colleagues should be considered carefully before being incorporated into the report. Once the details of content, organization, and style have been examined and revisions have been made, the report is ready to be printed in final copy.

Proofreading

The final copy should be scrutinized for any previously overlooked errors in spelling, punctuation, and grammar and compared with the rough draft to detect any omissions. The report should then be read aloud once more from beginning to end to check for organization, flow, and style (Theriault, 1971). Once the final corrections are made, the report is ready for signature.

Report Format

Nation and Aram (1977) believe that "clinical report writing should follow . . . the steps of the diagnostic process" (p. 330). According to Pannbacker (1975), a diagnostic report should be organized for easy retrieval of information. It also should reflect accuracy, completeness, clearness, conciseness, and prompt preparation (W. O. Haynes & Pindzola, 1998).

Using a standard format has several advantages: (a) it requires less time to write the report; (b) it helps ensure that all staff report similar information; and (c) it helps facilitate retrieval of information (Flower, 1984). Use of a standard format also may help new clinicians become familiar with the information contained in diagnostic reports. In some instances, it may be possible to use an abbreviated format designed for specific program needs.

According to Knepflar (1978), a weakness of some reports is that they provide information only about the major problems, and say nothing about other aspects of communication. If information is reported about each aspect of communication, the report serves as a baseline measure. It also helps to ensure that important information is not omitted.

Use of Sample Reports

There are many ways to learn to write reports. According to Meitus (1983), one way to learn report writing is to "read many samples of reports written by experienced professionals" (p. 297). It is helpful to have sample reports available for students, who can read the good reports and practice rewriting the poor ones.

The style and format of the report vary based on the specific purpose of the report, the setting in which the clinician works, the referral source, and the policies of particular facilities regarding report writing (Nation & Aram, 1977). Knepflar (1976) described several approaches to "tailor" reports to the needs of specific readers. Hanson (1979) indicated that if the report is carefully planned and written, it may provide necessary information for several reviewers.

Several sample reports representing different types and formats are provided in the appendixes. Complete reports on all disorders and all possible combinations are not reproduced because of space limitations. Other examples of reports and case studies are in texts readily available to speech–language pathologists (Blischak & Ho, 2000; Dalston, 1983; Dworkin & Hartman, 1988; Dworkin & Meleca, 1997; Hegde & Davis, 1995; Helm-Estabrooks & Aten, 1989; Lund & Duchan, 1988; Meitus, 1983; Middleton & Pannbacker, 1997; R. Miller & Groher, 1990; Nation & Aram, 1977; Shipley & McAfee, 1992; Stemple, 1993). Writers should review sample reports from a variety of other sources, including the facility in which they work.

The reevaluation report is written somewhat differently from the initial evaluation report. The date of previous evaluations should always be indicated in the reevaluation report, along with a brief discussion of initial evaluation findings and recommendations. History information should be updated at the time of the reevaluation. An example of a letter that may be used to request additional information from another agency or professional is provided in Chapter 4, Figure 4.2.

Current test results should be compared to the results of previous evaluations. Impressions and recommendations are based on all available information. The procedures for reevaluation are of particular interest to school speech–language pathologists, who must provide annual reviews of student progress.

The final step in the diagnostic report process is follow-up. The clinician must assure all paperwork and recordkeeping have been completed. Follow-up may be needed to determine whether the intended recipients received the report, whether the receiver understood or had questions about the contents, and whether the client has been seen for additional testing or is receiving treatment (W. O. Haynes & Pindzola, 1998). To avoid confusion, a letter like the one in Chapter 4, Figure 4.1, might accompany a report sent to the individual or facility that referred the client.

Types of Reports

A variety of diagnostic report formats have been utilized. It may be appropriate to use a general format, keeping in mind that reports vary based on the facility requirements and the intended receivers. Figure 2.1 provides an example of a standard (traditional) diagnostic report format that may be adapted to meet a variety of needs. A worksheet for following this format is provided in Figure 2.2. Sample standard reports are provided in Appendix A.

Facility-Based Formats

The Problem Oriented Medical Report (POMR) or Problem Oriented Report (POR) was originally designed for medicine but has been adopted for use by other health-care professionals, including speech–language pathologists. The POR system is based on a problem-solving process. It consists of (a) the database, (b) problem list, (c) plans, and (d) follow-up notes.

The database is a comprehensive compilation of initial information about an individual and the services received. It includes data about the individual's history, present problems, present life situation, results of previous speech–language evaluations, treatment notes, reports from other professionals or facilities, and correspondence (Bouchard & Shane, 1977; L. Kent & Chabon, 1980; Kettenbach, 1990; Peterson & Marquardt, 1994). Problems are identified, listed, and numbered. The resulting list serves as a table of contents and includes initial plans for treatment as well as a rationale for further evaluation (when appropriate), treatment plans, and client and family education.

Agency Identification (Letterhead)

Name: _____   Telephone: _____

Date of Birth: _____   Date of Evaluation: _____

Parents/Spouse (when appropriate): _____   Referral Source: _____

Address: _____   File Number: _____

e-mail address: _____

Speech and Language Evaluation

Statement of the Problem

Describe the problem. Identify the referral source and reason for referral. State where the information in the report was obtained.

History

Report information from referral letters, case history, and the parent/client interview. Report only pertinent information.

Examination

Summarize the findings of the evaluation, listing the tests used, their purpose, and the results. Use language that all receivers can understand. It may be helpful to briefly describe how the client responded and whether someone accompanied the client into the evaluation. Knepflar (1976) feels that the report should contain information about all aspects of the client's communication behavior. If a treatment plan must be written from the evaluation report, it is helpful to have specific information about what the client could and could not do.

Impressions

Summarize and integrate the information from the history and evaluation sections of the report. Report the diagnosis. Meitus (1983) feels that a diagnostic statement should contain "a disorder classification, a specification of the severity of the symptoms, a statement of the etiological and contributing factors, . . . factors that are expected to influence intervention . . . and a prognostic statement" (p. 296).

Recommendations

W. O. Haynes and Pindzola (1998) believe this may be the most crucial portion of the report. They note that this section is used to "translate our findings into appropriate suggestions or directions that will help the client solve communication and related problems" (p. 409). Recommendations should be specific and brief. They may include recommendations for treatment, parent training or counseling, reevaluation, and referral.

Signatures

Each signature should be followed by printed information including each examiner's name, title, and professional qualifications.

Figure 2.1. Standard (traditional) diagnostic report format.

The available data are analyzed and each speech–language problem is identified and listed. Problems may be symptoms, signs, instrumental findings, or combinations of factors that are associated with a specific speech–language disorder. Each problem is considered relative to (a) further evaluations needed, including a rationale; (b) treatment plans, including a statement of goals/objectives; and (c) client and family education, including the information necessary to understand the speech–language problem and their role in management. Problems are modified, added, or deleted as a function of new information or progress. The problem statement includes details such as the duration, frequency, severity, and current and past management of the problems.

Follow-up notes are entered in the client's record under the appropriate problem name and number. These notes may be in narrative form or flow sheets. All available client information

Sample Report Format Worksheet

Date: _____

Name: _____ Birthdate: _____ Chronological Age: _____

Parent(s): _____

Address: _____

Telephone: _____ Date of Evaluation: _____

File Number: _____

Speech and Language Evaluation

Statement of the Problem: _____

_____

History: _____

_____

Examination: _____

_____

Impressions: _____

_____

_____

Recommendations: _____

_____

_____

Signature(s) (Include Name, Title, ASHA Certification and State License)

_____

_____

_____

Figure 2.2. Worksheet for traditional or general report format.

is organized under four headings that form the acronym SOAP (see Table 2.11). The narrative form for the SOAP format includes Subjective data, Objective data, Assessment data, and the Plan for management.

Subjective data is information provided by the client or family, such as the symptoms and response to treatment (i.e., the interview and case history). Objective data includes observation by the clinician, test results, and information from referral sources. Assessment data provides the analysis, interpretations, and impressions including diagnosis by the clinician based on the subjective and objective data. The plan involves additional diagnostic testing, treatment, and client and family education. Information about PORs and SOAPs is also available elsewhere in the speech and language literature (Bouchard & Shane, 1977; Cornett & Chabon, 1988; Flower, 1984; Hays, 2000; L. Kent & Chabon, 1980; R. Miller & Groher, 1990).

Several advantages of the POMR/POR and SOAP formats have been identified, such as better communication with other professionals, better client management, better student training, and better record keeping (L. Kent & Chabon, 1980). Samples of problem-oriented reports are provided in Appendix B.

Integrated Diagnostic Reports

A general trend in treatment philosophy has been to treat the individual as a whole. This trend is seen in public schools beginning with Public Law (P. L.) 94-142, the Education for All Handicapped Children Act of 1975, which mandates that a child's entire educational program must be comprehensive and integrative. This trend is also seen in the medical environments, including rehabilitation centers and home health agencies, where a variety of professionals are caring for a client. Professionals providing assessment and treatment in areas of physical, cognitive, language, hearing, speech, and emotional functions provide a more comprehensive treatment program for a client. Some examples of integrated evaluation and treatment team professionals are the voice, stroke, cleft palate, hearing impaired, augmentative, and rehabilitation teams.

Team approaches to assessment and treatment require that professionals work closely together, and may require integrated reporting to document a client's overall function and progress. To provide for continuity of information and writing style, it may be preferable to assign one professional team member to compile the report. When an integrated diagnostic report is required, professional terms may need to be clarified or briefly defined within the report. Two examples of integrated reports are in Appendix C.

Treatment Plans and Reports

Treatment plans may form one section of diagnostic evaluation reports, or they may be separate reports (Flower, 1984).

Table 2.11
SOAP Format and Data

Term	Data	Description
Subjective	Interview	Patient's perception of something
		Case history experienced
		Interview generates more information about what the patient experiences
		Direct quote or summary of what the patient/family said
Objective	Test results	Data that can be perceived by the senses (seen, heard, smelled, felt); facts; reports from others
Assessment	Analysis or collation of subjective and objective information or data	Conclusion based on subjective and objective data; diagnosis
Plan	Additional testing and management options	What you plan to do next
		The next step in the teaching process (client and family education)
		Procedure for checking on patient/family compliance with the treatment regimen
		Date of next visit

Treatment plans should include long-term and short-term goals as well as statements about prognosis, and should specify the amount, frequency, and direction of treatment (ASHA, 1999f). The plans may be presented in outline or narrative form.

Client records should indicate when treatment plans were discussed with the client and family, and when conferences were held with other professionals to discuss treatment. Recommendations from the conferences should be included. Discharge recommendations and follow-up referral recommendations made to the client also should be noted in the client's record. According to ASHA's Professional Services Board (1999f), treatment reports should contain (a) the time period covered by the report, (b) the number and length of sessions, (c) the diagnostic summary, (d) the summary of the treatment plan, (e) the summary of the client's responses to the treatment plan, (f) the current client status, (g) the conclusions and recommendations, and (h) the signature and title of the qualified speech–language pathologist or audiologist who is responsible for the service.

Information about treatment is included in the POMR/ POR and SOAP formats. Cornett and Chabon (1988) described a flowchart format for treatment plans. The flowchart provides in a table format the objectives written in behavioral terms, procedures or techniques including the reinforcement method used to achieve each objective, and a written record of the results including stimulus items and the client's responses. Tonkovich (1989) described a format for using ASHA's Functional Communication Measures (FCM) in diagnostic reporting and treatment planning. The FCM format (a) improves time efficiency and cost effectiveness; (b) eliminates unnecessary details in reporting; (c) establishes uniformity in data collection and diagnostic nomenclature; (d) facilitates computer generation of reports; and (e) enables monitoring of quality assurance outcome indicators (Frattali & Lynch, 1989; Larkins, 1987). Nova Care (1989) also developed a format for functional outcome. The reporting of functional outcome is further discussed in Chapter 3. Examples of treatment plans are provided in Appendix D.

Individualized Education Programs (IEPs)

The Education for All Handicapped Children Act of 1975 (EHA) addresses education for children from 3 to 21 years of age. The Education of the Handicapped Act Amendments of 1986 (P.L. 99-457) ensured services for preschool children and created a comprehensive program for infants and toddlers (0–3 years) with disabilities. In 1990, EHA was renamed the Individuals with Disabilities Education Act (IDEA) (P.L. 101-476). Referred to as Part H, The Infant and Toddlers with Disabilities program, IDEA was amended again in 1991 to P.L. 102-119 (Myers-Jennings, 2000). These children must be identified, assessed, and educated in the most appropriate environment for each child's specific needs and abilities. The document that summarizes and correlates all of this information is termed an Individualized Education Program (IEP).

The IEP is a child-centered plan developed by the child's teachers, school administrators, remedial specialists, and parents. W. O. Haynes and Pindzola (1998) state that the IEP should respond to very specific questions: (a) What is the problem? (b) Where is the child functioning now? (c) Who will do what with the child and how often? (d) When and how is progress to be measured? Cornett and Chabon (1988) provide a checklist to assess and document the appropriateness of the IEP relative to legal requirements (includes all information required by law), relevance (objectives appropriate for student's diagnosis), manageability (reasonable criteria for time allotted to treatment), and clarity (comprehendible terminology and readily understandable outcome criteria).

Current practices provide that speech–language services be provided in a collaborative style in more inclusive educational settings such as classrooms. In addition, the treatment objectives are combined with the educational curriculum to make treatment objectives more relevant and functional to the child's daily living. In addition, the child's progress must be regularly reported. Reports must provide a description of the child's current level of performance along with a list of measurable annual treatment goals. Progress reports must be sent as often as indicators of educational progress are sent to parents of nondisabled children. Thus, progress reports are sent with report cards at the end of every reporting period. These regulations are required by the Individuals with Disabilities Education Act (IDEA) (U.S. Department of Education, 1999).

The specific format varies among school districts or state education agencies and it can range from simple to complex. Many school districts have simplified the procedure by using computer-generated formats that retain individuality of assessment and treatment plans but are more efficient than handwritten forms (Krueger, 1985). Nelson (1988) provides detailed individualized speech and language intervention programs for infants, children, and adolescents presenting a variety of disorders that are in accordance with EHA. Samples of IEPs are provided in Appendix E.

Some school-based speech–language pathologists also prepares the Individualized Family Service Plan (IFSP). The IFSP involves the assessment of the family as well as the child or student. Included in the IFSP report are (a) the child's current levels of development, such as cognitive, motor, speech, language, hearing, self-help, social, and behavioral; (b) the strengths and needs of the family in facilitating the child's development; (c) the expected outcomes for the child and the family; (d) the criteria and timelines for measuring progress; (e) the services needed to meet the needs of the child and family including their type and frequency; (f) the date treatment will begin and an estimated time period for the duration of the treatment; (g) the designated case manager; and (h) the procedures needed for the transition from early intervention into preschool (W. O. Haynes & Pindzola, 1998). A sample of an IFSP is provided in Appendix F.

Progress Reports

Progress notes, sometimes referred to as the daily log or working notes, should not be confused with progress reports. Progress notes usually are written immediately after each clinical session. These notes then serve as source material for periodic progress reports (C. Weiss, Lillywhite, & Gordon, 1987). Progress notes include (a) brief notes concerning specific clinical management techniques and materials used, (b) interpretation of how the client responded and statements regarding the client's progress, (c) suggestions or assignments given to the client, and when appropriate, (d) recommendations for the next clinical session (Knepflar, 1976). Notes are recorded in blue or black ink and signed by the clinician. Some practicing clinicians fail to keep daily progress notes, and others write abbreviated, incomplete notes that may be meaningful to them but of little value to anyone else (Knepflar, 1978).

Progress reports may be written for parents, referral sources, or cumulative files. Some insurance companies and most government sources of funding require periodic progress reports as a basis for continued funding. The style varies depending on the purpose, and the report may be very brief or rather detailed and data oriented. Reports to parents usually are in narrative form. Data-based progress reports for cumulative files are described by Simon and Holway (1985). A longitudinal evaluation summary is presented in a compact table format consisting of tests administered with the dates of administration and the child's chronological age at the time of each formal test administration. The percentages of responses for targeted communication skills at the time of each test administration are listed on the table adjacent to the test scores to show changes in test results and accompanying changes in communication skills, both in drill and conversation. This format provides a succinct display of scores for each formal test administration along with behavioral change data, thus showing the positive outcome of the treatment provided. Progress reports also may include information about specific clinical strategies that were helpful, those that were not helpful, or those that the client resisted.

The language of the progress report should be appropriate to the intended reader and written in objective terms that document changes in observable behaviors. A report to a parent that says, "Sarah is doing well in therapy and seems to enjoy working on her [s] sound," tells the parent nothing about Sarah's speech progress. A more acceptable sentence might read, "When reading single words beginning with [s], Sarah produces the [s] phoneme correctly in 90% of the words."

Discharge Planning and Reports

Good clinical practice involves discharge planning and the preparation of discharge reports (Flower, 1984). According to Duffy (1995), no treatment should begin without a plan about when it will end. At the beginning of treatment, a discharge plan developed and coordinated by the speech–language pathologist or audiologist should be prepared (Cornet & Chabon, 1988). Objectives of discharge planning are as follows:

1. To prepare the client and family for a change in or termination or services.

2. To help arrange a shift in care from one agency or professional to another.

3. To evaluate and identify current and anticipated communication needs.

4. To monitor the client's communication status following discharge.

5. To prepare the client and family to transfer acquired skills or techniques to settings external to the original place of treatment (Cornet & Chabon, 1988, p. 801).

Implementation of a discharge program usually involves several strategies:

1. the clinician assesses and diagnoses the severity of and prognosis for the client's communication problem;

2. the clinician formulates and implements a discharge plan to be followed by the client, family, or other healthcare providers based on the client's medical needs, family situation, transportation, insurance coverage, service options, motivation, and so on; and

3. the clinician evaluates the discharge plan through follow-up with the client, the family, and/or facility serving the client (Cornet & Chabon, 1988).

Discharge planning reports should contain the following information:

- Client identification information

- History

- Status at beginning of treatment

- Indications and contraindications to treatment

- Summary of treatment plan

- Number and length of treatment sessions

- Expected date for termination of service

- Discharge plan(s) including recommendations for whatever continued services and follow-ups are needed (Cornet & Chabon, 1988; Flower, 1984; Hegde & Davis, 1988; Kittenback, 1990)

Discharge reports should begin with a concise history of relevant services prior to the initiation of current treatment services (Flower, 1984). Next, the report should include speech, language, and hearing problems at the beginning of treatment. Finally, there should be specific discharge plans. If the problem-oriented medical record format is used, a discharge plan should be developed for each problem listed (Bouchard & Shane, 1977). Discharge reports usually should be sent to the original referral source, so the need for further services can be determined. Specific forms for discharge planning and follow-up can be found in Cornet and Chabon (1988).

Summary

Well-written evaluation reports are essential to speech–language pathology and audiology. Information gained from the evaluation is of little value until it has been documented in some usable form. In order to achieve a well written report, the clinician should follow the rules of writing through careful study of appropriate language usage, composition, form, and style.

Familiarity with the report writing process is essential to executing a well-written report. Steps involved in this process include planning, preparing, and writing the first draft; revising and refining the draft; and proofreading the final copy. Knowledge of a standard report format and study of sample reports are helpful in building report writing skills. The report process does not end with the signing of the initial report; follow-up and review are ongoing tasks and include reevaluation reports and a tracking process to assure that all paperwork has been completed within prescribed timelines.

There are several types of clinical reports: the traditional or standard report, Problem Oriented Medical Reports or Problem Oriented Reports, SOAP format, integrated diagnostic reports, treatment plans and reports, Individualized Education Programs, and progress reports. The format for reports is generally dictated by the work site. Regardless of format, all reports should provide objective and subjective data about assessment and treatment. Attention to clinical reports is important because they form the foundation for clinical services and establish the professional reputation of the clinician.

 Exercises

1. Interview a practicing speech–language pathologist or audiologist. Ask him or her to describe in detail the kinds of written reports required on the job. Write a brief report of your findings.

2. In a brief essay, identify and describe the kinds of professional writing that you expect to do. To whom will you be writing (colleagues, supervisors, clients, etc.)?

3. Compare the evaluation reports written in several different settings, noting the formats used, the length of the reports, the amount of detail included, and the types of recommendations made.

4. Why should simple, straightforward language be used when writing a diagnostic report?

5. Why are written reports essential to effective clinical practice?

6. Identify major barriers to effective report writing.

7. Review a diagnostic report from your clinic files. Without identifying the clinician, write a memo identifying the strengths of the report. Then, identify any weaknesses, and make recommendations for revision.

8. What are the advantages and disadvantages of using a standard report format?

9. Identify some of the potential problems associated with providing diagnostic reports to clients and their families. How can these problems be resolved?

10. Give reasons for using a standardized form to organize reports.

Reporting Outcome Data

Speech–language pathologists and audiologists in every practice setting are increasingly taking more of an interest in outcome measures. Recently the focus has been on the entire process of client care including diagnosis, treatment, discharge planning, and follow-up or after care (Cornett & Chabon, 1988). The use of outcome data to monitor the quality of speech, language, and hearing services has been advocated for many years but only achieved prominence in 1993 with the establishment of ASHA's Task Force on Treatment Outcomes and Cost Effectiveness. One of its projects was to invite recognized authorities to review the published information about treatment efficiency and provide reviews in eight areas of treatment: aphasia (Holland, Fromm, DeRuyter, & Stein, 1996), cognitive–communicative disorders (C. A. Coelho, DeRuyter, & Stein, 1996), dysarthria (Yorkston, 1996), hearing aids (Weinstein, 1996), hearing loss (Carney & Moeller, 1998), phonological disorders (Gierut, 1998), stuttering (Conture, 1996), and voice disorders (Ramig & Verdolini, 1998). The reports were published as supplements to two issues of the *Journal of Speech–Language and Hearing Research* in October 1996 and February 1998. Continuing with the activities of the Task Force, ASHA formed the National Center for Treatment Effectiveness in Communication Disorders (NCTECD) to coordinate outcomes and efficiency activities of the association. Since 1997 NCTECD has focused much of its efforts on the development and implementation of a National Outcomes Measurement System (NOMS) for speech–language pathologists working with children and adults in schools and healthcare settings (ASHA, 1998d, 1999c, 1999d).

ASHA's Scope of Practice in both speech–language pathology and audiology considers evaluation of outcomes. The "Scope of Practice in Speech–Language Pathology" (ASHA, 1996c) indicates that speech–language pathologists should "evaluate the effectiveness of their practices (and) modify services in relation to their evaluations" (p. 18). According to the "Scope of Practice in Audiology" (ASHA, 1996b), audiology services should be evaluated to determine "efficiency, cost benefit and consumer satisfaction" (p. 15).

ASHA's standards programs identify standards for outcome. The Professional Services Board (ASHA, 1999f) defines standards for clinical service in speech–language pathology and audiology. PSB Standard 3, quality improvement and program evaluation, states "the quality of services provided is evaluated and documented on a systematic and continuing basis; 3.1 there are written policies and procedures for evaluating the effectiveness and efficiency of client care and other key areas of program evaluation; 3.2 evaluation results are used to improve quality of care and program evaluation; 3.3 the evaluation process is reviewed and updated on a regular and systematic basis" (p. 12). The Council on Academic Accreditation (ASHA, 1998a) has several standards related to outcome. These standards are as follows:

5.2 The program has adequate physical facilities (classrooms, offices, clinical space, research laboratories) that are accessible, appropriate, safe, and sufficient to achieve the program's mission, goals, and objectives.

5.3 The program's equipment and educational/clinical materials are appropriate and sufficient to achieve the program's mission, goals, and objectives.

5.4 The program has access to clerical and technical staff, support services, and library and computer resources that are appropriate and sufficient to achieve the program's mission, goals, and objectives.

5.5 The program has access to a client base sufficiently large and diverse to achieve the program's mission, goals, and objectives and to prepare students to meet the ASHA recognized national standards for entry into professional practice. (p. 17)

ASHA's (1997b, 1997c) Preferred Practice Patterns consider outcome and documentation. "Outcomes of services should be monitored and measured in order to ensure the quality of services provided and to improve the quality of those services" (p. 9).

Review criteria are applied to a variety of data sources. The most common data sources are clinical and student records. Other sources include direct observation, interviews, questionnaires, and surveys. Assessments may be retrospective, concurrent, or prospective (see Figure 3.1 for related information). Retrospective studies or record audits are considered after the services are provided. Concurrent reviews are used to assess

---

Diagnostic Report Checklist

Use this as a guide to reviewing reports.

YES	NO	
☐	☐	1. Is the identifying information complete (name of client, date of birth, address, telephone number, etc.)?
☐	☐	2. Was the report ready on or before the due date?
☐	☐	3. Is the chronological age correct?
☐	☐	4. Are the complaint and referral sources identified?
☐	☐	5. Does your report follow a fully developed history, examination–impressions–recommendations structure?
☐	☐	6. Is only pertinent history information included?
☐	☐	7. Is the report written in correct standard English?
☐	☐	8. Is the information well organized and chronologically appropriate?
☐	☐	9. Do the impressions rest on the history examination?
☐	☐	10. Has the report been proofread?
☐	☐	11. Are all test results accurate?
☐	☐	12. Are all test results fully interpreted?
☐	☐	13. Does the impressions section contain only the essential information (nature and severity of speech–language–hearing problem, etiology, prognosis)?
☐	☐	14. Is the report in correct form?
☐	☐	15. Is the report free from grammatical errors?
☐	☐	16. Are the recipients of the report identified?
☐	☐	17. Is there consistency in use of present, past, and/or future tense?
☐	☐	18. Is the report concise?
☐	☐	19. Have unnecessary words, meanderings, and repetitions been eliminated?
☐	☐	20. Are recommendations for speech treatment, reevaluation, and follow-up included?
☐	☐	21. Are recommendations based directly on objective interpretation of data?
☐	☐	22. Is there a brief statement of recommendations given to the client or family for alleviation of the problem?

Each of the above questions should be answered Yes.
If you have answered No, revise that part of the report.

Figure 3.1. Diagnostic report checklist.

appropriateness of services as they are provided. Prospective reviews use established criteria to determine admission to a program (Cornett & Chabon, 1988).

Types of Outcome Data

Outcome data can be classified into peer review, consumer satisfaction, records audits, functional outcome measures, self-assessment and self-analysis, and financial data.

Peer Review

The essential concept underlying peer review is that the quality of services delivered by a professional is most appropriately assessed by peers in the same profession. Peer review can be used in medical or educational settings. The review should recognize local conditions and practices. According to Flower (1984), the concept of peer review is usually quite valid. Frattali (1992) stated, "Peer review has been advocated as the only possible form of quality control for clinical services, because it is said that only a practitioner's peers can judge his or her work" (p. 26). Centra (1979), however, questions the reliability of this concept because "colleague assessments may be distorted by mutual back scratching or by professional jealousy" (p. 73).

Occasionally, informal peer reviews involve a peer commenting to the clinician about clinical reports. Such opinions may not be representative and are probably less useful than those comprehensive or formal systems that ask peers for written responses to a set of preestablished criteria about clinical reports, such as those shown in Figures 3.1 and 3.2.

Some state associations and the Council of State Association Presidents have outcome-measurement projects (Harrison, 1998). These projects include member education, student education, efficacy, and payers.

Consumer Satisfaction

Consumer satisfaction measures are designed to obtain information about the quality of services from clients, families, or other consumer sources, referral sources, and students (Rao, Blosser, & Huffman, 1998). There are a variety of methods for surveying consumer satisfaction measures, as listed in Table 3.1. Several consumer satisfaction measures have been developed (Kreb & Wolf, 1997; Rao et al., 1998).

Chapey (1977) developed a 50-item consumer satisfaction questionnaire for speech–language pathology. ASHA's (1989) Consumer Satisfaction Measure (CSM) is a one-page questionnaire that addresses the degree of client satisfaction with timeliness of services, physical setting, interactions with staff, and service outcomes on a 5-point scale ranging from strongly disagree (1) to strongly agree (5) (Frattali, 1994; Rao et al., 1998). ASHA's (1989) Task Force on Treatment Outcomes and Cost Effectiveness developed a written client satisfaction questionnaire that uses a 5-point scale for each item (*strongly agree* to *strongly disagree*). The ASHA Subcommittee on Treatment Outcome Measures (1997d) developed a 9-item questionnaire about voice treatment outcomes that can be completed by clients, families, caregivers, teachers, or other listeners.

ASHA also has consumer satisfaction surveys, within each component of NOMS: birth to kindergarten (ASHA, 1996d), pediatric (ASHA, 1995b), and adult (ASHA, 1995d). Client satisfaction was high for skilled nursing facilities, rehabilitation hospitals, acute rehabilitation hospitals, and adults from all treatment settings.

Most consumer satisfaction surveys include only limited information about diagnostic reports. Figure 3.3 is an evaluation form that can be used for speech–language pathology or audiology reports. Obtaining specific information about reports is an important way of improving them (Ownby, 1987).

A limited number of studies have covered parents' perceptions of clinical reports. Watson and Thompson (1983) reported that 93% of parents indicated they understood the conclusion of written clinical reports. Earlier reports by Eisenstadt (1972) and Shipley and McCroskey (1978) suggest that

some parents believe that explanations of diagnostic findings are inadequate and inappropriate or that vague language is used by clinicians.

Reading level is an important factor in developing consumer satisfaction measures for clients and families. Illiteracy, which has been defined as reading skills below the fifth-grade level, is a major problem in the United States (Doak, Doak, & Root, 1985). Furthermore, individuals with communication problems and their families are more likely to have reading problems.

Student evaluation is an important aspect of measuring consumer satisfaction. Evaluation of speech–language pathology and audiology graduates is a requirement for accreditation from ASHA's Council of Academic Accreditation (CAA). The CAA requires a comprehensive evaluation plan of the quality and effectiveness of the professional performance of a training program's graduates for at least a 5-year period. Other aspects of the consumer satisfaction assessment process include students' evaluation of the quality of academic and clinical training. Most students have an opportunity to comment on strengths and weaknesses of a course or clinical practicum experience, and sessions to improve the course or practicum. In addition, students are asked to rate the class or practicum and teachers or supervisors at the end of each semester. There are no global measures of consumer satisfaction for students; it is common for training programs to develop their own consumer satisfaction measures to be considered during the training period, at the end of the training program, and following training.

Records Audits

Records audits are used by different people for different purposes. They may be conducted by external agencies, such as accreditation committees, or they may be internal audits conducted by administrators, peers, or the persons providing the services (Flower, 1984).

Records audits or review of records are used in both clinical and academic settings. There are several guidelines that govern methods of assessing and reporting outcome by reviewing records of clients or students. These guidelines include Preferred Practice Patterns (ASHA, 1997b, 1997c), Scope of Practice (ASHA, 1996b, 1996c), and Council on Academic Accreditation (ASHA, 1998a). Forms for audits in health care and academic clinical training programs are shown in Figures 3.4 to 3.7.

Functional Outcome Measures

The need for functional outcome data has been emphasized by Campbell (1999a, 1999b, 1999c) and Frattali (1998). Several measures have been developed for assessing and reporting functional communication outcomes. Sarno (1965, 1969) introduced the *Functional Communication Profile* for individuals with aphasia. Forty-five items related to movement, speech,

Worksheet for Clinical Reports

Client ID: _____ Clinician: _____

Reviewer: _____ Date: _____

Rating Scale

1 = Unsatisfactory   4 = Good, More than Adequate

2 = Fair, Less than Adequate   5 = Excellent

3 = Average, Adequate   X = Unable to rate or not appropriate

_____ Met deadline for report

_____ Knew when, how to deviate from routine format for reports

_____ Provided accurate and complete identifying information

_____ Organized information well; chronologically appropriate

_____ Indicated purpose of evaluation

_____ Clearly identified source of information

_____ Reported impressions including nature and severity of communication problem, etiology, and prognosis

_____ Made accurate and complete recommendations

_____ Provided information appropriate for intended recipient

_____ Reported history information and test results accurately

_____ Included supplemental client and/or family observations

_____ Exercised caution in making statements outside of profession

_____ Integrated information

_____ Made appropriate recommendations and/or referrals

_____ Used direct quotations when appropriate

_____ Used accurate grammar, punctuation, and spelling

_____ Demonstrated knowledge and appropriate use of terminology

_____ Was concise

_____ Avoided criticism of other professionals/agencies

_____ Overall rating of report

Comments _____

_____

Figure 3.2. Worksheet for clinical reports.

Table 3.1
Methods of Surveying Consumer Satisfaction

Questionnaire Format	Administration
Multiple-choice questions	Mail
Yes/No questions	Telephone
Rating scales	Manual distribution and immediate return
Open-ended questions	Face-to-face interview
Time Frames	**Client Tracking**
Retrospective	Anonymous
Concurrent	Identified by name
Prospective	Coded
	Identified by program
Frequency of Use	**Responsibility for Gathering Data**
Continuous	Administration
Monthly	Communications/Media relations
Quarterly	Outcomes management/Program evaluation
Intermittent/Sporadic	Consumer affairs
	Quality improvement
Subject Sample	Separate clinical department
All discharged clients	
All clients receiving services	
Random sample	
Stratified random sample	

Note. From "Measuring Consumer Satisfaction," by P. R. Rao, J. Blosser, and N. P. Huffman, 1998, in *Measuring Outcomes in Speech–Language Pathology*, by C. M. Frattali (Ed.), New York: Thieme. Copyright 1998 by Thieme. Reprinted with permission.

understanding, and reading are rated on a 9-point scale from *poor* to *normal*. Holland (1980) developed the *Communicative Abilities in Daily Living* first for use with adults with aphasia and later for use with adults with mental retardation, Alzheimer's disease, and hearing aids. ASHA designed functional communication measures for children and adults that are based on a 7-point scale from *normal* to *profound*.

Self-Assessment and Self-Analysis

Flower (1984) believes that "the only truly effective approaches to quality assurance depend upon professionals monitoring the services they provide" (p. 321). McCarthy (1990) feels self-assessment measures are ideal quality assurance measures. Several approaches to self-assessment or self-analysis of clinical reports are available. One approach involves reviewing and rewriting clinical reports after completion of the original clin-ical report. Another approach uses a structured format, such as a self-appraisal form, for reviewing clinical reports. The format is similar to that used for peer reviews and records audits in Figures 3.1 and 3.2.

Financial Data

Outcome data is critical to speech–language pathology and audiology, but an analysis of financial outcome may be mandatory for survival of the professions (Rolnick & Merson, 1998). Both clinical and financial outcome data should be collected and reported. Clinical outcome data alone is not enough—cost effectiveness must be determined. There are several systems for collecting and analyzing financial outcome data. The Functional Independence Measure is a multidisciplinary scale that includes demographic and financial data. The Beaumont Outcome Software System (Merson, Rolnick, & Weiner, 1995)

(text continues on p. 49)

Evaluation of Speech–Language and/or Audiology Reports

We are attempting to determine how well our reports meet the needs of persons who request speech–language and/or audiological assessment. This questionnaire is designed to provide information about the extent to which the evaluation report provided the information you requested. Your feedback is important in helping us improve the quality of our services. The first seven items can be answered by checking the appropriate response to each question. The other questions are designed to provide feedback about other aspects of the report.

1. Does this report answer your referral questions(s)? ☐ Yes ☐ No ☐ Partially

2. Was the report clear and understandable? ☐ Yes ☐ No ☐ Partially

3. Does this report provide new information or insights? ☐ Very helpful ☐ Somewhat helpful ☐ Not helpful

4. Does this report confirm the insights that you already had about the client? ☐ Very much ☐ Somewhat ☐ None

5. Is the information provided in this report helpful in developing new ideas about helping this client? ☐ Very helpful ☐ Somewhat helpful ☐ Not helpful

6. Does this report provide useful recommendations about treatment methods that may be appropriate for this client? ☐ Very useful ☐ Somewhat useful ☐ Not useful ☐ None provided

7. What is your overall evaluation of this report? ☐ Highly helpful ☐ Somewhat helpful ☐ Not helpful

8. What type of information did you request when you referred this client for a speech–language and/or audiological evaluation?

   ☐ eligibility for speech–language services ☐ suggestions for speech–language treatment

   ☐ information to increase your understanding of the client ☐ other (please specify) _____

9. What, if any, additional information should have been included in this report?

   _____
   _____
   _____

10. What, if any, information from the report will be useful in your work with this client?

   _____
   _____
   _____

11. What, if any, of the recommendations for this client will you implement?

   _____
   _____
   _____

12. What, if any, suggestions can you provide to help the examining speech–language pathologists and/or audiologists improve their reports?

   _____
   _____
   _____

13. Please indicate your position (if appropriate):

   ☐ physician ☐ client

   ☐ teacher ☐ special education teacher

   ☐ counselor ☐ administrator/supervisor

   ☐ speech and language clinician ☐ other (please specify) _____

   ☐ family of client

Figure 3.3. Form for evaluation of speech–language and/or audiology reports.

Health Care Facility Chart Audit

Facility Name: _____

Month: _____

Resident Name	Initial Eval. Page 1 & 2	Monthly Follow-up	Care Plan	Daily/ Weekly Notes	D/C Summary	Orders			D/C Care Plan	MD Cert. (Part B only)	Comments
						I	C	D			

Signature: _____

Date: _____

Figure 3.4. Health care facility chart audit. *Note.* D/C = Discharge, I = Initial, C = Clarification, D = Discharge.

Audit for Student Files

Program: _____   Department: _____   Date: _____

Student Name	Application	UG Transcript	GRE	Rx Letters	A & R Letter	Accept Letter	ASHA Course Breakdown	Academic Program	Transcript	Observations	Clinic Clock Hours	Clinic Evals

Signature: _____   Date: _____

Figure 3.5. Audit for student files. *Note.* UG = Undergraduate, GRE = Graduate Record Examination, Rx = Recommendation, A & R = Admissions and Review.

Audit for Speech–Language Services

Treatment: _____ Semester: _____ Date: _____

I = Incomplete   C = Complete   N = Not Needed

Student Name	Release	Log	Fee	Reduction	Eval. Report	Progress Report	Rx	FCM	Comments

Continue _____ Dismiss _____ Audit _____ Discharge _____

Signature: _____ Date: _____

Figure 3.6. Audit for speech–language services. *Note.* Rx = Recommendation, FCM = Functional Communication Measure.

Client Folder Audit

Reviewer: _____

Date: _____

Type of Review: ☐ Diagnostic   ☐ Treatment

Period of Review: _____

Student Name	Supervisor	History Intake	Info. Released	Fee Reduction	Log	Following	FCM	Evaluation Report	Progress Report	Comments

Signature: _____   Date: _____

Figure 3.7. Client folder audit. *Note.* Log = Chronological of all services provided, FCM = Functional Communication Measure.

can be used to collect clinical and financial outcome data as well as client satisfaction. ASHA's outcome measures (1995b, 1995c, 1996a) also allow for collection of data about clinical and financial data, and client satisfaction.

Assuring Quality of Documentation in Health Care Facilities

Assuring the quality of documentation is an important aspect of outcome and is related both to functional and financial outcomes. One of the most frequent causes of denials of payment for services is based on what the intermediary terms "a lack of skilled services" or a determination that the "services of a skilled therapist were not required." Written documentation is the only review source on which the intermediary can base those conclusions. Therefore, it is critical that the clinician responsible for treatment or documentation be alert to requirements for documenting that services were "skilled."

Skilled speech–language pathology services must meet all of the following conditions:

- Services must be necessary for the diagnosis and treatment of speech–language disorders which result in communication disabilities or for the diagnosis and treatment of swallowing disorders (dysphagia), regardless of the presence of a communication disability.

- Services must be related directly and specifically to a written treatment plan established by the physician after any needed consultation with the speech–language pathologist.

- Services must be reasonable and necessary to the treatment of the individual's illness or injury.

- Services must be considered under accepted standards of practice to be a specific and effective treatment for the patient's condition.

- Services must be of such a level of complexity and sophistication or the patient's condition must be such that the services required can be safely and effectively performed only by or under the supervision of a qualified speech–language pathologist.

- There must be an expectation that the patient's condition will improve significantly in a reasonable and generally predictable period of time based on the patient's restorative potential assessed by the physician or the need to establish a safe and effective maintenance program related to a specific disease state.

- The amount, frequency, and duration of the services must be reasonable.

The documentation system for health care serves three major purposes: as a medical legal record, as a mechanism for justification for reimbursement, and as a communication tool to internal team members (i.e., nursing staff, practitioners in other disciplines, physicians).

Additional reasons for health care documentation include consistent professional terminology to describe patient status and treatment, and less possibility of duplication of services between treatment disciplines. As for guidelines, supportive documentation should exist between disciplines, any changes or emphasis in treatment must be reflected in weekly notes, and documentation should show that the client has restorative potential.

Table 3.2 compares skilled and nonskilled procedures commonly found in medical speech–language pathology.

For documentation to support coverage of speech–language pathology services, that documentation should include an objective component that is compared to previous reporting and demonstrates progress toward a stated functional goal.

▶ **Example:** Achievement of 75% of word naming compared to last month's score of 50%. (Note that these percentages should be based on real numbers, i.e., 75 out of 100.)

To carry this further, the functional goal should include information about the word-naming task that is necessary for the client to improve "functioning" in his or her environment. For example, the word-naming task might reflect vocabulary related to clothing worn frequently by the patient, food items the patient likes and dislikes, and names of familiar persons in his or her life. Naming of kitchen items might be irrelevant and viewed as nonfunctional if the patient is not now or in the future going to function in a kitchen.

Documentation using narrative statements should also contain reference to objective scoring and comparison of previous scores or the treatment plan with present status compared to previous status. The following are examples of narrative statements that would not support coverage for speech–language services:

- "Mr. Jones is very concerned about going home. He was having difficulty with family again today." (no comparative or objective data)

- "Speech is somewhat slurred today." (vague and subjective)

- "Mr. Jones achieved 75% accuracy on word-naming tasks." (no comparative data and no functionality)

- "Mr. Jones has shown significant improvement in his ability to make himself understood." (vague and subjective with no supporting data)

Figures 3.8 to 3.10 provide guidelines for documentation of treatment plans.

Table 3.2
Comparison of Skilled and Nonskilled Procedures

Skilled Procedures

1. Diagnostic and evaluation services to ascertain the type, causal factors, and severity of speech and language disorders. Reevaluation if the patient has a change in functional speech or motivation, clearing of confusion, or remission of some other medical condition which previously contraindicated speech pathology services.

2. Evaluation and diagnosis of the speech, language, or any related disorder.

3. Design of a treatment program relevant to the patient's disorder. Continued assessment of the patient's progress during the implementation of such treatment program, including documentation and professional analysis of patient's status at regular intervals.

4. Establishment of a hierarchy of tasks and cueing that directs a patient toward communication goals.

5. Establishment of compensatory skills (e.g., air-injection techniques, word finding strategies) and analysis related to actual progress within the goals.

6. Selection and establishment of augmentative or alternative communication devices.

Nonskilled Procedures

1. Nondiagnostic/nontherapeutic routine, repetitive and reinforced procedures (e.g., the practicing of word drills without skilled feedback).

2. Procedures that may be repetitive or reinforcing of previously learned material that staff or family may be instructed to repeat.

3. Procedures that may be carried out by any nonprofessional (e.g., family member, restorative nursing aide) after instruction and training are completed.

4. Provision of practice for use of augmentative or alternative communication systems.

Summary

There are several types of outcome data that speech–language pathologists and audiologists should know about. These include peer review, consumer satisfaction, records audits, functional outcome measures, self-assessment and self-analysis, and financial data. Assuring the quality of documentation is related both to functional and financial outcomes.

 Discussion Questions

1. How has ASHA advocated for the development and implementation of outcome data?

2. Why has the reliability of peer review been questioned?

3. What is the difference between formal and informal peer reviews?

4. Describe methods for assessing consumer satisfaction.

5. What ASHA guidelines can be used to develop records audits?

6. How can functional outcomes be assessed?

7. What systems are available for collecting functional outcome data?

8. How is documentation related to both functional and financial status?

Plan of Treatment for Patient Rehabilitation

☐ Part A Medicare ☐ Part B Medicare ☐ Other Complete at end of first month of treatment for initial claims only.

1. Patient Last Name (as on Medicare card) Patient First Name		2. Provider Number	3. Health Insurance Card Number
4. Provider Name (facility name)	5. Medical Record Number	6. Onset Date	7. Start of Care Date
8. Type ☐ PT ☐ OT ☐ SLP ☐ CR ☐ RT ☐ PS ☐ SN ☐ SW	9. Primary Diagnosis (pertinent medical dx)	10. Treatment Diagnosis	11. Visits from Start of Care

12. Plan of Treatment Functional Goals
   Goals (Short-term)

   1–4 week measurable goals
   functionally oriented
   related to long-term goals

Outcome (Long-term)

Patient function and status expected at time of discharge from your department

Plan

Treatment modalities and procedures
Educational plan
Equipment/products plan
Discharge plan

13. Signature, Professional Designation (of person establishing plan of care)

14. Frequency/Duration (e.g., 3/wk × 4 wk)

   frequency (no range), BID?, Duration to meet LTG

I certify the need for these services furnished under this plan of treatment and while under my care. ☐ N/A

15. Physician signature   16. Date

17. Certification
   From   Through   ☐ N/A

18. On File (print/type physician's name)

19. Prior Hospitalization
   From   Through   ☐ N/A

20. Initial Assessment (History, medical complications, level of function at start of care)

Reason for Referral:

Evaluation information
   Prior and pertinent medical history, complications, contraindications—Medical necessity
   Previous functional status: where, with whom, assistive devices, what activities
   Current functional level/deficits
   Reason for skilled therapy services
   Prognosis for rehabilitation goals you've established
   Patient's goals

NOTE: Onset date listed in section #6 must relate to the reason for therapy. If onset was greater than 6 months prior, state why services are needed at this time.

21. Functional Level (at end of billing period) Progress Report   ☐ Continue Services   OR   ☐ Discontinue Services

At End of Month:
   Compare initial status to end of month functional status.
   Document why there has not been significant change if that is fact (i.e., only 2 visits so far; medication change altered patient's cognition). Balance, etc.: patient has had UTI, etc. If patient is discharged prior to end of first month, discharge summary should be written here. Include comparison of status, number of treatments, status of goals identified, discharge location, and plan for further intervention on continuum of care.

22. Service Dates:
   From   Through

Figure 3.8. Plan of treatment for patient rehabilitation.

Updated Plan of Progress for Patient Rehabilitation

☐ Part A Medicare ☐ Part B Medicare ☐ Other   Complete at end of first month of treatment for initial claims only.

1. Patient Last Name (as on Medicare card) Patient First Name	2. Provider Number	3. Health Insurance Card Number
4. Provider Name (facility name) 5. Medical Record Number	6. Onset Date	7. Start of Care Date

8. Type ☐ PT ☐ OT ☐ SLP ☐ CR ☐ RT ☐ PS ☐ SN ☐ SW | 9. Primary Diagnosis (pertinent medical dx) | 10. Treatment Diagnosis | 11. Visits from Start of Care

12. Frequency/Duration (e.g., 3/wk × 4 wk)

13. Current Plan Update, Functional Goals (Specify changes to goal and plan goals)
(Short-term)
Updated measureable
1-to-4 week goals
Functional
Related to long-term goals
If not changed, document why in #18

Outcome (Long-term)
LTGs as before, unless changed. If changed, document why in #18

Plan

Updated treatment modalities and procedures
Education plan
Equipment/products plan
Discharge plan

(If changed, document why in #18)

I certify the need for these services furnished under this plan of treatment and while under my care. ☐ N/A

14. Certification   From   Through   ☐ N/A

15. Physician signature   16. Date

17. On File (print/type physician's name)

18. Reason(s) for Continuing Treatment This Billing Period (Clarify goals and necessity for continued skilled carer.)

State why patient needs continued skilled therapy services. Should relate to treatment plan and goals. Don't just reiterate problem list, but relate deficits, complications, positive prognostic indicators, etc., as they relate to function and long-term goals!

Demonstrate your clinical judgment process.

Justify any changes in treatment plan and goals. (Does nursing documentation support this justification?) Use skilled terminology.

19. Signature, Professional Designation (of person establishing plan of care) | 20. Date | 21. ☐ Continue Services ☐ Discontinue

22. Functional Level (at end of billing period). Relate your documentation to functional outcomes and list problems still present.

Compare this section at end of 2nd month. If physician has not yet returned the original, write your note on the copy in the medical record and document on the original, when returned, to see attached copy.

Compare prior end of month functional status to current month functional status, listing problems still present requiring your skills.

Document any barriers or complications to meeting goals—that is, patient illness, medication change, symptoms of depression (don't write "patient depressed" as a diagnosis), and any other complications that hindered progress. State your justification for ability to progress patient to meet goals.

23. Service Dates: From   Through

Figure 3.9. Updated plan of progress for patient rehabilitation.

Updated Plan of Progress for Patient Rehabilitation

☐ Part A Medicare   ☐ Part B Medicare   ☐ Other   Complete at end of first month of treatment for initial claims only.

1. Patient Last Name (as on Medicare card)	Patient First Name	2. Provider Number	3. Health Insurance Card Number
4. Provider Name (facility name)	5. Medical Record Number	6. Onset Date	7. Start of Care Date

8. Type ☐ PT ☐ OT ☐ SLP ☐ CR ☐ RT ☐ PS ☐ SN ☐ SW	9. Primary Diagnosis (pertinent medical dx)	10. Treatment Diagnosis	11. Visits from Start of Care

12. Frequency/Duration (e.g., 3/wk × 4 wk)	

13. Current Plan Update, Functional Goals (Specify changes to goal and plan goals) (Short-term) Were STGs upgraded? Are they measurable and functional? If unchanged, is there justification in #18? Outcome (Long-term) LTGs as before, unless changed. If changed, document why in #18	Plan Were these changes in the treatment plan from last month?

I certify the need for these services furnished under this plan of treatment and while under my care. ☐ N/A	14. Recertification From Through ☐ N/A
15. Physician signature 16. Date Is doctor's signature (MED B) dated prior to recertification date?	17. On File (print/type physician's name)

18. Reason(s) for Continuing Treatment This Billing Period (Clarify goals and necessity for continued skilled carer.)

Do you understand why goals were not met? Do you understand why they were upgraded? Has any change in frequency and duration been explained to your satisfaction? Is it clear why therapy is going to be continued? Does the reasoning make sense to you? Is skilled terminology used?

19. Signature, Professional Designation (of person establishing plan of care)	20. Date	21. ☐ Continue Services ☐ Discontinue

22. Functional Level (at end of billing period). Relate your documentation to functional outcomes and list problems still present.

Is the patient's functional level addressed and compared to beginning of month? Can you identify improvement?

Is there a justification for lack of improvement in patient function and a reasoning process evident for why we should expect the patient to have improvement and meet goals in the very near future?

23. Service Dates: From   Through

Figure 3.10. Updated plan of progress for patient rehabilitation.

Clinical Correspondence

Correspondence with clients, families of clients, and professionals is an important clinical activity (Hegde, 1998). Speech–language pathologists and audiologists write many different kinds of documents: referral letters, appeal of denials for funding, letters of recommendation, nomination letters, memos (memoranda), and resumes. Copies of all correspondence should be maintained (Cornett & Chabon, 1988). Each document generally has a specific format and contains certain kinds of information (Berger, 1993).

The typical focus of graduate training in speech–language pathology and audiology is on writing diagnostic reports, treatment plans, and clinical outcome summaries. Students are not usually taught very much about writing letters and memos. Only limited information about clinical correspondence in speech–language pathology and audiology is available (see Cornett & Chabon, 1988; Hegde, 1998; Hegde & Davis, 1999; Roth & Worthington, 1996). This chapter discusses some of the more important kinds of letters and memos, provides suggestions about writing them effectively, and describes the formats for each kind of correspondence in some detail.

Referral Letters

Correspondence related to referral issues provides documentation for record keeping and is an important professional activity (Roth & Worthington, 1996). There are three types of referral letters: (1) those written to acknowledge referral of a client, (2) letters describing treatment progress, and (3) letters making a referral to another professional. Examples of Types 1 and 3 are in Figures 4.1 and 4.2. Information about progress reports written as letters can be found in Hegde (1998) and Hegde and Davis (1999).

Letters of Recommendation

It is not uncommon to be asked to write letters of recommendation for students or peers. Letters of recommendation for students are usually related to job application or admission to graduate schools. These letters should include the following:

- courses or clinical experiences the student had with you, whether the student was a clinical trainee or student employee, and how long you have known the student

- performance of the student in your courses or under your supervision, specific papers the student wrote, projects completed, and his or her contribution to class discussions

- intellectual qualities and character of the student and a comparison of the student with other students you have taught or supervised

- prediction for the student's future success in graduate school or in professional work (Berger, 1993)

Mentioning race, religion, ethnicity, age, and any related matters should be avoided. To mention these matters would be a violation of ASHA's (1994a) Code of Ethics Provision IV, Rule F, which states, "individuals shall not discriminate in their relationships with colleagues, students, and members of allied professions on the basis of race or ethnicity, gender, age, religion, national origin, sexual orientation, or disability" (p. 2).

Many facilities provide forms on which to write answers to specific questions about applicants. It may be helpful to write a "To Whom It May Concern" letter for the student, which addresses the topics listed earlier. This has two advantages: (1) it reduces the delay in the student's obtaining letters of recommendation and (2) it reduces the number of letters the instructor or supervisor needs to write for the student.

Keith-Spiegel, Wittig, Perkins, Balogh, and Whitley (1993) described a number of issues related to writing reference letters for students. These issues include the negative letter, biasing, hurt feelings, and previous and insider information. The authors provide solutions for problems related to these issues.

It is not unethical to include negative information about a student in a recommendation letter; however, the data upon which the information is based must be specific and honest (Keith-Spiegel et al., 1993). Berger (1993) believes it makes sense to be honest and realistic, mentioning a student's deficiencies and weaknesses, as well as strengths. It is generally impossible for a student to have high ratings in every area.

(text continues on p. 58)

B. S. Jones, M.D.
56151 Main Street
Shreveport, LA 71135

Dear Dr. Jones:

Thank you for referring Jane Johnson (4 years, 6 months of age) to the Speech and Hearing Center at Smith State University for a speech and language evaluation. Jane was seen for this evaluation on August 5, 2001. She was accompanied by her parents, who were concerned about her lack of understandable speech.

Results of the evaluation revealed a mild to moderate speech and language delay. Jane's speech was characterized by a reduced repertoire of phonemes, the omission of phonemes, and errors in producing both vowels and consonants. Single-word articulation was better than articulation in connected speech. Her receptive language or understanding far exceeded her ability to communicate orally. Jane passed an audiometric screening.

It is recommended that Jane receive treatment for her speech and language problems at the nearest available speech–language center. Enclosed is a copy of her speech and language evaluation report. If you have questions or concerns about this report, please feel free to contact me.

We appreciate your referral and look forward to continued collaboration with you.

Sincerely,

Joe B. Backer, M.S., CCC-SLP

Figure 4.1. Referral acknowledgment.

Joe B. Smith, M.D.
Director, Cleft Palate Team
Jones State University
Shreveport, LA 71135

Dear Dr. Smith:

Sammy Chavez, a 6-year-old boy, is being referred to the Cleft Palate Team for direct examination of velopharyngeal closure. Sammy was seen for a speech and language evaluation on August 10. His speech was characterized by hypernasal resonance and nasal emission, and weak pressure in the production of the pressure consonants.

Sammy has a history of nasal regurgitation and has been in a speech treatment program for 2 years focusing on nonspeech oral motor exercises to reduce hypernasality and to improve velopharyngeal function; progress has been poor.

A copy of the evaluation report is enclosed along with the parents' written authorization for the release of this information. Please send me a copy of your examination report. Call me if you have questions about this client. I appreciate your help.

Sincerely,

S. S. Katz, M.S., CCC-SLP

Figure 4.2. Referral letter.

Where there are specific weaknesses, it is appropriate to mention them; this strengthens the credibility of the writer and suggests a fair evaluation of the student. The importance of the deficiencies should be assessed, followed by a description of what, if anything, the student is doing about them. Weaknesses can be minimized somewhat by focusing attention on the student's strengths and special areas of expertise.

Resumes

A resume is a summary of a person's background, experience, training, and skills (ASHA, 1999b; Coxford, 1987). A resume should be accompanied by a cover letter. If possible, one should indicate the specific position applied for and source of information about the position (Mahmoud, 1992). Examples of cover letters can be found in Beatty (1984), Cole and McNichol (1997), Coxford (1987), and Dickhut (1987).

Common Myths About Resumes

There are several myths and misconceptions about resumes. It is important to be aware of these myths to avoid developing a resume that could be detrimental to professional viability. The most commonly held myths are as follows:

▶ **Myth #1:** Resumes should never exceed one page in length. Kennedy (1998) refers to this as "the one page or bust resume" (p. 264).

  Truth: Resumes should be of reasonable length but long enough to adequately describe experience and professional qualifications (Beatty, 1984).

▶ **Myth #2:** Longer resumes describe qualifications better and are more effective.

  Truth: Resumes of unreasonable length could make it difficult, if not impossible, to determine an individual's most significant qualifications and accomplishments.

▶ **Myth #3:** Unique or unusual resumes attract attention and are better read.

  Truth: Although unique or unusual resumes may attract attention, they are often viewed with a high degree of suspicion. Rather than conveying an image of originality, creativity, or intellect, most unusual resumes raise red flags that the individual may be a nonconformist, a loner, or an eccentric.

▶ **Myth #4:** Resume content is more important than style or format.

  Truth: Poorly written or disorganized resumes suggest that the individual may be insensitive, inconsiderate, sloppy, disorganized, confused, uninformed, undisciplined, or worse.

▶ **Myth #5:** An individual can exaggerate accomplishments because nobody checks resumes.

  Truth: Sooner or later exaggerations or misrepresentations will be discovered and be embarrassing (Beatty, 1984). Kennedy (1998) calls this "the fibs are fine myth" (p. 265).

▶ **Myth #6:** Listing references is important and conveys "solid" character.

  Truth: This is no longer an encouraged resume practice; it could signal that one is not up to date with current practices.

▶ **Myth #7:** Listing hobbies and extracurricular activities is important and conveys the image of a diversified, well-rounded person.

  Truth: Modern resume concepts typically exclude hobbies, which take up space on the resume that could be used more effectively to describe qualifications or work-related achievements. Only two situations warrant inclusion of hobbies on the resume: (1) if they are directly job related and (2) if a person is applying to a facility that is known to place a high value on such activities.

▶ **Myth #8:** Indirectly, one's status as married conveys a mature or stable image.

  Truth: There may be little to be gained from including marital status on the resume. Beatty (1984) recommends that women eliminate it altogether.

▶ **Myth #9:** Personal photos improve resume appearance and enhance marketability.

  Truth: Most employers are intolerant of those who include a photograph with their resume. Including a personal photograph suggests that the individual is out of touch with current practices.

▶ **Myth 10:** Use of salary history on a resume can enhance favorable salary treatment and demonstrates salary progression.

  Truth: Salary history or current salary should not appear on the resume. There are several reasons for excluding salary information on the resume: (a) it is considered to be in poor taste, (b) employers are not interested in salary-related promotions, (c) it may give the impression of being "money hungry" or of having a shallow value system, and (d) premature disclosure of salary or salary requirements may automatically eliminate one from consideration or be less than what might be offered.

▶ **Myth #11:** Cover letters are better read than resumes.

  Truth: Resumes are considerably more important, and are usually much better read than the cover letters that accompany them.

▶ **Myth #12:** The functional resume is the most effective format.

Truth: This type of resume summarizes major accomplishments and achievements at the beginning of the resume. Some shortcomings of the functional resume are that it is often used by those who have something to hide, and it is considerably more difficult to read and comprehend than the chronological format (Beatty, 1984).

▶ **Myth #13:** The resume can be prepared in 90 minutes.

Truth: Thinking that a resume can be written in 90 minutes or overnight is ridiculous. Good resumes take time and effort (Kennedy, 1998).

▶ **Myth #14:** The typewriter will do.

Truth: The difference between computer printouts and typewriter-produced pages is obvious. Computer produced resumes suggest that one is up to date and able to handle word processors (Kennedy, 1998).

▶ **Myth #15:** The resume does it all.

Truth: The resume is only one market tool in a job search that can result in an interview (Kennedy, 1998).

▶ **Myth #16:** The resume is to blame.

Truth: Maybe yes, maybe no. Telephone calls and interviews may also be factors (Kennedy, 1998).

▶ **Myth #17:** You can always expect an answer.

Truth: Prospective employers may not acknowledge receiving a resume (Kennedy, 1998).

▶ **Myth #18:** One type of resume is sufficient.

Truth: One may need more than one type of resume (Kennedy, 1998).

Resume Preparation

Suggestions for preparing a resume include the following:

1. Use standard-sized paper.
2. Make it visually appealing and easy to read.
3. Keep comfortable margins with clear and organized sections.
4. Make space breaks between paragraphs and sections.
5. Use capital letters, indentations, or underlining to set off words and names.
6. Check and recheck for typos, misspellings, and smudges.
7. Send photo-offset or original (first-copy) documents.
8. Keep the format simple.
9. Do not copy someone else's resume. You want your resume to be about you, not someone else.
10. Be honest and factual.
11. Use action words.
12. Avoid the use of pronouns.
13. Be specific in your job descriptions and spell out your accomplishments.
14. Incorporate phrases rather than complete sentences—phrases are short and "punchy" and work better.
15. Avoid gimmicks like fancy lettering and bright-colored paper (white, gray, and beige are "safe" colors).

A resume should be carefully reviewed after it is compiled, and revised as necessary. A rating sheet for preparing resumes is presented in Figure 4.3.

Resume Formats

The three basic resume styles are (a) chronological, (b) functional, and (c) hybrid or combination (Kennedy, 1998). The chronological resume is the most traditional and frequently used type of resume (Cole & McNichol, 1997). It lists employment in reverse order with current or last employment shown first (Dickhut, 1987). An advantage of a chronological resume is that it demonstrates professional growth, and is straightforward and easy to follow (Cole & McNichol, 1997). Disadvantages are that it highlights job changes and periods of unemployment and deemphasizes skills acquired in various settings by location in different parts of the resume. The functional format is ability focused and divides responsibilities or achievements by work functions or classifications. Advantages of a functional resume are that it (a) focuses on skills and competencies not reflected in recent job history and (b) is adaptable to special circumstances such as lack of direct experiences or difficult to explain job gaps or changes. Disadvantages of a functional resume are that (a) it must provide a clear professional objective and (b) it may give the impression of hidden information (Cole & McNichol, 1997). The hybrid is a combination of reverse chronological and functional formats.

Other formats for resumes include the curriculum vitae, portfolio, electronic or digital, and Internet. The curriculum vitae is a comprehensive summary of professional employment, education, honors, memberships, and scholarly achievements such as grants, publications, and presentations (Kennedy, 1998). The portfolio format consists of samples of work organized in a portfolio. The electronic or digital resume is similar to a traditional resume in that it is a record of education and

---

Checklist for Resumes

Include comments as to how an area could be improved. Rate the resume based on the following scale:

	1 = Excellent	2 = Satisfactory	3 = Needs Work

Area	Score	Comments / Improvements
Overall appearance	_____	_____
Readability	_____	_____
Layout	_____	_____
Consistency	_____	_____
Length	_____	_____
Relevance	_____	_____
Writing style	_____	_____
Action-oriented	_____	_____
Specificity	_____	_____
Employment	_____	_____
Education	_____	_____
Accomplishments	_____	_____
Completeness	_____	_____
Effectiveness	_____	_____
TOTAL	_____	

Score

14–17   Current resume is excellent; do not make unnecessary changes

18–21   Good resume; target areas for improvement; work on making it better

22+   Need to reevaluate the resume as it is now, and revise it

Figure 4.3. Checklist for resumes. *Note.* From *Revising Your Resume* (pp. 151–152), by N. Schuman and W. Lewis, 1987, New York: Wiley. Copyright 1987 by John Wiley and Son. Reprinted with permission.

---

experience. Its content and format are designed to be compatible with a computer (Weddle, 1998). The Internet resume is designed to be transmitted from any computer to any other computer on the Internet or on the World Wide Web. It uses a format called American Standard Code for Information Interchange (ASCII). There are several advantages of high-tech resumes: speed, accuracy, cost savings, flexibility, starting point, and a value-added credential of having knowledge of the Internet and its capabilities (Weddle, 1998).

Resume Contents

The contents of a resume depend, in part, on the type of resume and on personal preference. The content for a recent

graduate in speech–language pathology or audiology should be organized into categories, such as identifying information, personal data, professional objective, education, professional experience, clinical practicum experience, community service/volunteer work, professional memberships, honors and awards, publications, presentations, special skills, and references. After a clinician has obtained ASHA's Certificate of Clinical Competence, the clinical practicum experience should be eliminated. Table 4.1 lists information that should never be included in a resume. For further information about resume contents, refer to ASHA's (1999b) *For Life After Your Graduate School*, Anthony and Roe (1998), Beatty (1984), Bloch (1997), Cole and McNichol (1997), Coxford (1987), Criscito (1997), Dickhut (1987), Fournier and Spin (1999), Grapp and Lewis (1998),

Table 4.1

Information That Should Not Be Included in a Resume

Health or physical description

Race, sex, age, or national origin

Marital status or information about children

Religion or church affiliation

Political preferences

Photographs of self

Salary (current or desired)

The words "resume," "fact sheet," or "curriculum vitae" as a title

References (provided on a separate sheet if requested)

Written testimonies

Pronouns such as I, we, and they

Note. From *Tools for a Successful Job Search*, by P. A. Cole and J. G. McNichol, 1997, Rockville, MD: American Speech-Language-Hearing Association. Copyright 1997 by ASHA. Reprinted with permission.

Kay (1997), Kennedy (1998), Schuman and Lewis (1987), and Weddle (1998).

Resources for Resumes

There are two resources for assistance with resumes: professional resume writing services and software and online help. Professional resources are more than clerical services. They provide specialized knowledge about writing and producing resumes. Several software programs are available as well: *Win-Way Resume, Web Resume, Tom Jackson Presents the Perfect Resume,* and *Resume Maker* (Kennedy, 1998). The Internet has resume writing professionals online.

Nomination Letters

There are different kinds of nomination letters: letters of recommendation for promotion and for honors and awards. This kind of letter writing is important but generally not taught. The content of a nomination letter should clearly communicate the significance of the person's professional qualifications and contributions. Examples of these letters are presented in Figures 4.4, 4.5, and 4.6.

Memos (Memoranda)

The memo is the basic communication form used in most organizations. A memo is a short written communication that is used for interoffice communication of rules, policies, procedures, announcements, and other information (Berger, 1993; Mahmoud, 1992). A standard memo has five parts: "To," "From," "Date," "Subject," and the content of the memo (Mahmoud, 1992).

Appeals

Speech–language pathology and audiology services are sometimes denied by medical and insurance providers. Speech–language pathologists and audiologists need to know how to appeal the denied services. The format for an appeal letter is in Figure 4.7. Examples of denial statements for appeals are in Figure 4.8. Another resource for appealing denied insurance claims is the *Appeal Letter,* a free online newsletter (net.news, 1999).

Summary

Speech–language pathologists and audiologists write many different kinds of clinical correspondence. This includes referral letters, letters of recommendation, resumes, nomination letters, and memos. Each type of correspondence has a specific format and contains certain kinds of information.

 ## Discussion Questions

1. What kinds of correspondence do speech–language pathologists and audiologists write?

2. What information should be included in letters of recommendation?

3. Why are letters of recommendation addressed "To Whom It May Concern" useful?

4. How should weaknesses be addressed in letters of recommendation?

5. How can myths about resumes be detrimental?

6. Why should salary history including current salary not be included in a resume?

7. What type of resume would you prepare? Why?

8. Describe the advantages of high-tech resumes.

April 8, 2001

Mark Donald, Ph.D.
Eastern State University
Speech Pathology and Audiology Program
Durant, OK 74701

Dear Dr. Donald:

It is a great pleasure to support the nomination of Dr. Robert Thomas for the DiCarlo Award for clinical achievement. I first met Dr. Thomas in 1974 when he entered the University of Jamestown as a doctoral student in speech–language pathology. Since then, we have presented workshops about differential diagnosis of language disorders in children, voice disorders, and professional issues such as licensure and supervision. Most recently, I chaired the session he presented on the autism spectrum at the annual meeting of the Louisiana Speech-Language-Hearing Association in Baton Rouge. His presentation was to an audience of almost 400; he received a standing ovation.

Dr. Thomas is nationally recognized and respected as a clinical researcher in the area of autism. He has consulted about clients with autism and presented lectures and workshops throughout the United States. He is truly an exceptional clinician who has made a major contribution to the diagnosis and treatment of autism.

While it is primarily Dr. Thomas's clinical achievement that I believe warrants his nomination for the DiCarlo Award, his effectiveness as a teacher should not be overlooked because through his excellence in this area he has also made lasting contributions to the clinical training of speech–language pathologists. It is not only students but colleagues who learn from him.

I am pleased to support Dr. Thomas's nomination for the DiCarlo Award.

Sincerely,

M. P. Chang, Ph.D.
Professor and Program Director

Figure 4.4. Nomination for award.

August 26, 2001

Carmen Rodriguez, M.A., CCC-SLP
Chair, Professional Education Committee
P.O. Box 308
El Paso, TX 78218

Dear Ms. Rodriguez:

Robin Moore, a second-year student in the graduate program at El Paso University, is the unanimous choice for the scholarship from the Texas Speech-Language-Hearing Association (TSHA). Among the reasons are:

Overall GPA
    Texas A&M University at Bryan 3.98
    El Paso University 4.00

Financial
    In addition to tuition and book costs, com-
        mutes 150 miles per day to attend classes
    (Current state rate per mile = 0.28) = $840.00
        per month)

TSSLHA membership and participation
    Texas A&M University at Bryan, secretary
        1997 to 1998
    El Paso University, President 1998 to Present

Honors or recognition
    Texas A&M University at Bryan, summa cum laude
    El Paso University Student of the Year, 1998 to 1999

Community Service
    Youth Leadership Leader, 1997 to 1998
    Vacation Bible School Teacher, 1996 to 1997
    Central Association for Retarded Citizens, 1993 to
    1995

Future professional plans
    Provide speech–language services in an underserved
    rural area

Robin is a dedicated student who works beyond maximum requirements; that is, she is truly exceptional. She has a positive, pleasant attitude and, in spite of the 150-mile drive, is often the first student to arrive in the morning and the last to leave in the evening. It would be difficult if not impossible to find a graduate student more deserving of the TSHA scholarship than Robin Moore. She is the student unanimously selected by the faculty as a nominee.

Sincerely,

_____
Pamela Parker, Ph.D.
Professor & Program Director

_____
Gustavo Morales, Ph.D.
Associate Professor

_____
Joyce Estrada, Ed.D.
Associate Clinical Professor

_____
James Frederick, Ph.D.
Associate Professor

_____
Connie Hayes, M.S.
Assistant Clinical Professor

_____
May Wood, M.A.
Assistant Clinical Professor

_____
Jennifer Cole, M.A.
Instructor

Figure 4.5. Nomination for scholarship.

October 10, 2001

Thomas Rubenstein, Ph.D.
Professor and Chair
University of Shreveport
Communication Sciences & Disorders Department
2919 Shreveport Avenue
Shreveport, LA 71104

Dear Dr. Rubenstein:

This letter is in response to your request of September 19, 2001 that I review Dr. Jean Carrazco's curriculum vitae relative to her qualifications for promotion to the rank of Professor in the Department of Communication Sciences and Disorders at the University of Shreveport (US).

Dr. Smith's curriculum vitae documents her progress toward meeting the criterion for promotion to full professor at US including (1) superior achievements and continued excellence in academic endeavors; (2) national or international recognition, and (3) comparable stature with others in the same rank and discipline at other peer institutions.

Particularly noteworthy are Dr. Carrazco's record of scholarly achievement in the area of grants and service. She has been the recipient of several grants; the total amount of these grants is more than one million dollars ($1,130,000). Dr. Carrazco has devoted considerable time and effort to serving on departmental, college, and university committees. From 1996 to 1998, Dr. Carrazco has served on an average of 10 committees per year. In addition, Dr. Carrazco served as Program Director (May 1994 to July 1996) and Coordinator (July 1996 to present).

Dr. Carrazco is an outstanding teacher. She has been nominated and has received teaching awards in 1987, 1988, 1992, and 1996. She has also developed computer assisted instruction and has presented this information at state and national workshops including the annual meeting of the American Speech-Language-Hearing Association in 1989, 1991, 1994, and 1996.

Dr. Carrazco has published 20 papers in scholarly journals including the *Journal of Communication Disorders* and the *Journal of Speech and Hearing Research*. In addition, she is a co-author of three chapters in a book, *Clinical Research in Speech–*

Figure 4.6. Letter for promotion.

Page 2

Language Pathology and Audiology, which was published by Uptown Press. Dr. Carrazco has also presented 40 papers and workshops at professional meetings such as the American Speech-Language-Hearing Association (1989, 1991, 1992, 1994, 1997).

In summary, Dr. Carrazco's curriculum vitae suggests that she be given timely consideration for promotion to the rank of professor.

Sincerely,

Mary Pannbacker, Ph.D.
Professor

Figure 4.6. Continued.

TO: *Intermediary*

FROM: *Name of Facility*

DATE:

SUBJECT: Denial of Medicare Services for _____ (patient)

HIC#: _____

Period of Denial: _____ to _____

Claim Determination Letter Dated: _____

Reason for referral: _____

_____

Why were skilled services needed? _____

_____

   Medical necessity: endurance, bed mobility, transfers, ambulation, strength

Document need for skilled services during course of treatment:
   As shown in evaluation and recertification.
   As shown in weekly progress notes.

Close appeal letter with statement encouraging the reviewer to contact you if needed and thank the reviewer.

Therapy short term: only 3 weeks.

Figure 4.7. Format for appeal letter.

Examples of Denial Statements for Appeals

Dates of service: 09-01-99 to 09-03-99

Denial for speech–language pathologist—enough time has elapsed to establish a maintenance program.

Speech–language pathologist was necessary to teach and train caregivers in the follow-through of the functional maintenance program. Prior to this date, the patient's performance with oral feeding and safety has improved, and patient increased in his independence in follow-through. Caregivers, including the patient's son, need training in monitoring and prompting patient for clearing his mouth between bites and alternating liquids and solids. The training was essential to continue the swallowing safety that the patient has gained.

Dates of service: 07-01-00 to 07-31-00

Denial for speech therapy—enough time has elapsed to establish a maintenance program.

Skilled speech intervention was required during the denial period due to the patient's high risk of aspiration. Trial oral feedings began on 07-14-00. Primary method of nutritional intake (PEG tube feedings) continued. Despite amount of food consumed, patient continued to experience difficulty with oral intake. On 07-27-00 he was having a nonproductive cough, and pooling along with pocketing. These signs could result in premature spillage into the lungs. Normal airway protective mechanisms are diminished as a result of the CVA; this is evident by the lack of a productive cough(s). He was unable to utilize compensatory techniques effectively to reduce the risk of aspiration. At one time during the denial period, respiratory therapist was required to a conduct a lung assessment as a result of pooling and coughing. Continuous tube feedings were changed to bolus feedings when oral intake was under 75% on 07-08-00. Skilled intervention was warranted to continue to train the resident in utilizing these strategies to reduce the risk of aspiration.

Figure 4.8. Examples of denial statements for appeals.

Computerized Report Writing

Revision of reports typed on a typewriter requires time-consuming retyping, sometimes of several drafts. With the increased availability of electronic equipment, writing, revising, and changing report formats are less arduous tasks because they can be accomplished without retyping the entire report. In addition, computers can provide more efficient interpretation of test data and can manage clinic files and data for rapid retrieval.

Despite the availability of laptop computers, some writers find writing by hand on a tablet more portable because a power source is not needed. Of course, one reason may be limited typing skills. However, the deciding factor may be whether one can compose while typing (Henson, 1999).

Word Processing

The capabilities and flexibility of word processing software make it a powerful tool for report writing. The simplest word processors permit typing the first draft of a document, saving it on disk or hard drive, printing it out, and making as many revisions as necessary. Some people prefer to make revisions on a hard copy, and then enter these revisions in the computer document. Others choose to work with the document on-screen. Any changes are "invisible" in the final document (Berger, 1993).

Because word processing provides the opportunity to focus on writing, revising, and editing instead of on retyping drafts, it has become widely used. Many programs can merge data into previously designed report templates (Smith, 1993). Word processing software significantly decreases the time spent in report writing because errors, including spelling, can be corrected prior to printing the final draft. It is important to remember that a spell checker can find only misspelled words, not words used incorrectly (Henson, 1999). Scored test results or history information can be entered, then edited, rewritten, and reorganized into a different sequence later. Standard paragraphs entered into memory can be used to reduce typing time (Cohen, 1984; Silverman, 1987). The features of word processing can increase the writer's efficiency by organizing each document quickly and easily.

Individualizing Formats for Reports

Each clinical setting has a recommended format for reports that generally contains similar information placed in different sections. Repetitive items can be stored, then copied and edited each time a report is generated. Using "typeover" and "insert" modes, the current date, identifying client data, and information relevant to referral, history, examination, impressions, and recommendations can be entered under the appropriate headings. See Figure 5.1 for an example of a report format created for reporting the results of speech–language evaluations.

Specialized Software and Applications

Software is available that can simplify report writing for diagnostic evaluations and for Individualized Education Programs (IEPs). Table 5.1 provides the names and sources for currently available software. Because technology evolves so rapidly, however, additional resources may become available or those listed may become unavailable. Catalogs are the best source for the latest information. It is important when considering report writing software to evaluate the quality of reports as well as their applicability for each individual clinical circumstance. Sample reports are available and should be evaluated and reviewed prior to purchase.

There are even word processing programs that do not require use of a keyboard to input information. One example, *Naturally Speaking Preferred*, is listed in Table 5.1. Being able to draft a report by speaking into the computer instead of typing may be useful for individuals with poor typing skills, and it may be a faster way to fashion reports.

Computerized Interpretation

Since time and expertise are costly, practitioners must examine all options that can reduce expenses (Smith, 1993). One such option is computerized interpretation of test data. Some tests with computerized interpretation of results are listed in Table 5.2. Again, current catalogs may reveal additional resources as this is a fast-changing area. Speech–language

---

Speech–Language Evaluation

Insert and replace information where appropriate in this format. After proofreading carefully, use the spell-checking feature before printing the final copy.

Date: _____

Name: _____   Telephone: _____

Birth date: _____   Evaluation date: _____

Parents: _____   Referral: _____

Address: _____   ICD–9 Code No.: _____

This ___-year-old was seen for a speech–language evaluation at the Speech and Hearing Center on _____. This client was referred by _____.

Reason for referral: _____

Background information: _____

_____

Evaluation: _____

_____

Impressions/Findings: _____

_____

Recommendations: _____

_____

Evaluator's name: _____

Title: _____

License/Certification information: _____

Figure 5.1. Report shell for reporting speech–language evaluation.

---

pathologists in the future may be able to use the computer to administer and score a test, integrate results with other tests, and send the data to a report writing program for final editing and development of recommendations (Flynn, Parsons, & Shipp, 1999).

Computerized interpretation requires careful consideration (McCullough, 1990). Scoring time can be reduced significantly, with reduction of calculation errors; however, the clinician must still apply professional judgment, weighing mitigating assessment circumstances. Table 5.3 provides an overview of issues to consider.

Data Reports

The focus of this chapter has been on writing client reports. However, data reports are also important in speech, language, and hearing services. These include fiscal information, clinical activities reports, hearing aid inventories, and clinic schedules. The capability of the computer to handle and summarize data can simplify data reporting.

Reports of program evaluation can be generated by the computer. One example is the Beaumont Outcome Software System (BOSS), available from Parrot Software, P.O. Box 250755, Bloomfield, MI 48325. This software's reporting functions include comprehensive tables, charts, and graphs to illustrate outcome and cost.

Compiling databases on computers permits collection of large data sets of outcome information, which can be used to guide professional practice and policy development and refine funding decisions of third-party payers. In 1995 ASHA's Task Force on Treatment Outcomes and Cost Effectiveness announced the development of a treatment outcomes database for the professions (ASHA, 1995b). The first reports detailed information collected with adults in 100 health care settings (ASHA, 1996a). Additional studies are planned to reflect the

Table 5.1
Commercially Available Software To Assist with Report Writing

Software	Source	Description
Wordweaver Report Writing Software	Data Morphosis 118 South Ridge St., Ste. 196 Rye Brook, NY 10573 www.datamorphosis.com 914-939-4507	Answers to questions are compiled into a diagnostic report
Diagnostic Report Writer: Children	Parrot Software P.O. Box 250755 West Bloomfield, MI 48325-0755 www.parrotsoftware.com 800-727-7681	Based on answers to questions, reports are generated for children 2 to 16 years of age wih communication disorders
Instant IEP and Report Writer	Parrot Software (see above)	Selects wording to use with the data provided
The IEP Companion Software (accompaniment to IEP companion)	LinguiSystems, Inc. 3100 4th Avenue East Moline, IL 61244-9700 www.linguisystems.com 800-760-4332	Clinician chooses individual and classroom objectives for speech and language
Phonetic Font Plus	Parrot Software see above	Contains a subset of the International Phonetic Alphabet (IPA) to describe misarticulations
Naturally Speaking Preferred	Dragon Systems 320 Nevada St. Newton, MA 02470 www.academic-software.com 800-433-6326	Creates, edits, and revises documents by voice (hands free)
The Speech & Language Report Writer™	Clinician's Magician, LTD P.O. Box 426 Bedford, NY 10506 www.cliniciansmagician.com	Individual and classroom goals and objectives for speech and language Generates reports, organizes database for quick retrieval (free trial period provided) Contains a library of many phrasings to avoid similarities between reports

Table 5.2
Commercially Available Software To Assist with Interpretation of Test Results

Software	Source	Description
Clinical Evaluation of Language Fundamentals–Third Edition (CELF–3)	Communication Skill Builders/ The Psychological Corporation 555 Academic Court San Antonio, TX 78204-2498 www.psychcorp.com 800-872-1726	Generates norm-referenced scores and a narrative report which can be attached to an IEP
Automatic Articulation Analysis Plus	Parrot Software P.O. Box 250755 West Bloomfield, MI 48325-0755 www.parrotsoftware.com 800-727-7681	72 picture stimuli; Clinician records responses by clicking phonetic symbols; Analysis immediately available
Parrot Easy Language Sample Analysis Plus	Parrot Software (see above)	Elements of language sample presented in manner to clarify grammatical strengths and weaknesses of the speaker

Table 5.3

Issues To Consider in Computerized Interpretation

Advantages	Disadvantages
Scoring may be more consistent and accurate. Retrieval of norms may be facilitated. Overall errors are decreased.	Data entry errors can still be a problem.
Computerized interpretation programs are neutral with respect to biasing factors such as academic and social abilities, socioeconomic status, ethnicity, and race.	Equipment or trained personnel may be difficult to find. Training time may be prohibitive, and priorities for equipment usage may have to be established.
Scoring time is reduced significantly.	A scoring program that is current when purchased will need updating over time. A means of updating products previously sold and removing outdated products from the market need to be included in any marketing plan.
The computer can act as a memory aid in interpreting multi-scale tests.	
Moderator effects (i.e., age groups or ethnic groups with different ranges or patterns of scores) can be included in computerized interpretation.	It remains the professional's responsibility to maintain final authority over interpretation of results.
Profile analysis and statistical processing are impractical to implement with a hand-scoring method. Further, hand scoring has a high probability of calculation errors. Computerized scoring programs easily do the calculations and present interpretations of results.	Using the computer to preserve practices that have historical basis justifying existence requires debate and careful examination.
Computerized interpretation lessens the burden of writing repetitive, detailed descriptive content to educate those who read reports.	The use of computerized interpretations does not absolve the professional of applying clinical judgment. Reservations and mitigating assessment circumstances must be weighed independent of the computerized interpretation.
Language that is reasonably understandable may be ensured by careful development of narrative within the computerized program.	

Note. Adapted from Schrank (1994) and C. S. McCullough (1990).

clinical activities of all aspects of speech–language pathology and audiology services provided across all settings and populations (ASHA, 1995b).

Electronic Reporting

As e-mail becomes an increasingly popular way to send information, using it to report on clients is tempting. Some precautions are in order. E-mail tends to be somewhat informal and may be written too hastily. Once it is sent it cannot be retrieved and may not be as private as desired. E-mail may be stored in back-up files in servers that can be accessed by others. Because e-mail is so convenient, it may lead to information overload. If using e-mail to communicate client information, compose the document carefully as a file, look it over, think about it, and then send it (Berger, 1993).

Fax machines can also be used to send already written memos, letters, or reports almost instantaneously to anyone in the world. Confidentiality may be an issue depending on who monitors and distributes the incoming faxes.

Procedures for Managing Records

A. Schwartz (1986) and Koller (1986) stress the need to develop procedures for protecting the confidentiality of client records by controlling access to them. Security measures may include safe, secure storage of diskettes holding client information or specific access codes for entering client files in a hard drive or mainframe system. The problem of ensuring security while maintaining easy retrieval and use must be considered. If precautions are taken, security and confidentiality should be at least as easily monitored when using a computer system as when using hard-copy files.

Summary

The agony, frustration, and pain of report writing have been eased significantly by word processing and other computer programs. The report format used by individual clinic settings can be programmed and special reports can be organized and printed without being retyped. Client data can be compiled faster, more easily, and more accurately than ever before, using compatible word processing and database software. Computers can help professionals do their jobs with greater efficiency. They can also be used creatively to change and improve services as the use of computerized assessment, treatment, and management of outcome data increases (McCullough, 1990).

 Exercises

1. If you are interested in some of the applications described in this chapter, use a word processor to write to the suppliers for additional information.

2. If you have access to word processing and use it regularly, how would you feel about going back to a regular typewriter? Share your answer with someone who has never used a computer.

3. What are the limitations of using a computer for report writing?

4. Do you know a speech–language pathologist who is using a computer to generate reports? List the applications used.

5. Indicate whether the software applications listed above have been modified to serve specific needs of the program.

6. Review current catalogs to find report writing software. Request a sample report and evaluate it.

7. Find tests that offer computerized interpretation. Evaluate the advantages and disadvantages of computerized interpretation for your applications.

Reading and Writing Clinical Research Reports

CHAPTER 6

For speech–language pathologists and audiologists, reading and writing clinical research reports are important means of acquiring new information and improving clinical practice and treatment decisions. Reading research reports has relevance for all speech–language pathologists and audiologists, not only the minority who actually do research. Skill and efficiency in reading and writing clinical research reports increase with training and experience, although this area is not usually given significant emphasis in clinical training.

Reading Clinical Research Reports

Readers differ; they have their own preconceptions and interests. The major differences are among those who read for diversion, those who want a solution to a problem, and those who pursue knowledge and understanding (Booth, Colomb, & Williams, 1995).

Critical reading is necessary because clinical research reports vary considerably in the quality of speech–language pathology and audiology research. Publication is no guarantee of quality; both good and inadequate or marginal reports are published. Readers must therefore be prepared to identify weaknesses and limitations in published reports.

The validity of published reports and the applicability of validity to clinical practice are important. Knowing how to critically review and use clinical reports is imperative for optimal client care. Unfortunately, some speech–language pathologists and audiologists believe all published reports are reliable and become victims of bad products and faddish claims (Hegde, 1994). As Ventry and Schiavetti (1986) point out, "to modify and improve clinical services, scholarly practitioners must be able to evaluate critically the research literature relevant to their clinical practice" (p. 21). Pullum (1991) believes that the scholars should be immune or at least resistant "to uncritical acceptance of myths, fables, and misinformation" (p. 159).

Reasons for Critically Reviewing Published Reports

Speech–language pathology and audiology reports are critically appraised for a variety of reasons. First, published information must be critically reviewed if it is to be applied in making clinical decisions. Second, evaluating published reports is an important component of continuing professional development; it is essential for the professional who wants to meet the challenges of an ever-changing profession (Doehring, 1988). Third, scholarly activity and research can be facilitated through critical reviews of published reports (Baldwin, Goldblum, Rassin, & Levie, 1994). Fourth, critically reviewing published reports can provide valuable practice to both students and professionals. Students are often required to prepare critiques of published reports to demonstrate mastery of methodological and analytical skills (Polit & Hungler, 1991). Practicing professionals are sometimes asked to write critiques of manuscripts to assist editors in making publication decisions or to accompany a paper as published commentaries.

Quality of Published Reports

Another major reason for critically reading published reports is the tremendous variation in the quality of published information. Polit and Hungler (1991) believe "there is a tremendous range in the quality of reports, from nearly worthless to exemplary" (p. 584). According to Kuzma (1984) "it is a well-known, but regrettable, fact that some research literature is of poor quality. After wading through a mire of jargon, inconsistencies, poor grammar, tangles of qualifications, and some muddy logic, the user is expected to draw a brilliantly clear scientific conclusion. This problem is chronic in much scientific writing" (p. 224). Venolia (1987) feels that "slipshod writing breeds distrust," and promotes "readers to wonder if language is the writer's only area of incompetence" (p. 2). Ventry and Schiavetti (1986) caution that the appearance of an article in a journal is no guarantee of quality. There are good articles, and there are poor articles, both of which may be published. R. B. Haynes, Mulrow, Huth, Altman, and Gardner (1996) state that "many studies at all stages are flawed or reported misleadingly" (p. 1).

The quality of published research is affected by reliability, validity, design, and peer review. Understanding these concepts can ensure fewer difficulties for readers in critically reading reports. Reliability, the repeatability or constancy of data, is influenced by the size of the sample, the control of the variables, and the precision of the measures (Shearer, 1982). Validity means the degree to which a measurement device measures what it purports to measure, in other words, the appropriateness of the observations for answering the questions they are used to answer. Two areas of validity should be considered: internal validity and external validity. Internal validity refers primarily to the control of experimental variables and elimination of extraneous factors that would bias the results of a study (Shearer, 1982). Extraneous factors include gender differences, age, subject fatigue, socioeconomic status, intelligence quotient, and environmental conditions. External validity refers to how well the study relates to the real world. Factors that could influence external validity include sample size, selection of subjects, use of control groups, and interpretation of the findings. Fink (1998) provided specific guidelines for evaluating reliability and validity.

Readers should determine whether an appropriate design was used for the study. Using appropriate designs influences the truth of the information generated from statistics. Each design has different strengths and weaknesses (Coury, 1991). Polit and Hungler (1991) described specific guidelines for reviewing research designs. The major deficiencies of design are inadequacies related to definition, control, answering the question, neglect of important measurements, unimportant outcome measures, and biases (Kassirer & Campion, 1994). Fink (1998) developed a checklist for evaluating the quality of research design.

Peer review is a form of quality control. Editors of professional journals use reviews of manuscripts by peers with relevant expertise to select the papers to be published (ASHA, 1991–1992). Peer-reviewed journals are considered superior to non–peer-reviewed journals because of their expert scrutiny and the likelihood that serious errors will be detected and eliminated (ASHA, 1991–1992). Reviewers are instructed by the editor to prepare written evaluations that identify defects of originality and accuracy, comment on omissions and weaknesses, and point out deficiencies in writing style (C. R. King, McGuire, Longman, & Carroll-Johnson, 1997; Macrina, 1995). Manuscripts are accepted or rejected on the basis of reviews, or reviewers may recommend that the author revise and resubmit the paper. In 1997, the rejection rate of articles submitted for publication in the *Journal of Speech, Language, and Hearing Research* averaged 49% and ranged from 20% to 70% depending on the number submitted (Gordon-Salant, 1998).

It may be helpful to consider other factors related to the quality of a published report. The primary test of a publica-

tion's importance is the extent (if any) to which it modifies clinical practice (Lundberg & Williams, 1991). Additional factors such as readership, citation, and peer review are identified in Table 6.1. Citation counts of the number of times an author's publications are cited in subsequent literature are considered to be one of the more objective indicators of quality (Centra, 1979). However, it frequently takes up to two years for a manuscript to be published, and a few years after that before citations are published and can be indexed.

There are other reasons for critically reading published reports. One reason is the inaccuracy of references and quotations. Errors are common because many authors do not verify references and quotations (Benning & Speer, 1993; Goldberg et al., 1993; Hinchcliff, Bruce, Powers, & Kipp, 1993; Nuckles, Pope, & Adams, 1993).

Another reason for critically reviewing the literature is that statistical errors are not uncommon (Colditz & Emerson, 1985; Pocock, Hughes, & Lee, 1987). Findley (1990) described mistakes such as "use of standard error of the mean instead of standard deviation with skewed data, failure to describe the statistical tests used, multiple comparisons, and failure to use special forms of the test and χ^2" (p. 205). Ottenbacher (1995) pointed out that "there appears to be considerable confusion regarding the distinction between reliability (consistent) and agreement (consensus)" (p. 177). Thus, clinicians and researchers may be misinterpreting the statistical results of reliability investigations.

Guidelines for Critical Review of Published Reports

Critical review of publications is very different from recreational reading and often requires multiple rereading (Meltzoff, 1998). Critical analysis of published reports involves a careful appraisal of both strengths and limitations. Both adequacies and inadequacies are objectively identified in a good review (Polit & Hungler, 1991). Critiques should not be confrontational or degrading, but should provide constructive criticisms and may even provide evidence to support the views expressed (Portney & Watkins, 1993). Critical appraisal of published reports is a skill that requires background knowledge about research, theory, and clinical practice (Doehring, 1988; Portney & Watkins, 1993). There are several strategies for learning to critically review published reports. These strategies include published guidelines, knowledge of common deficiencies in the literature, training, participation in journal groups, reviews of the literature, and ability to generalize the impact on clinical practice.

Published Guidelines

In the past 10 years, guides have been created to aid in the critical appraisal of published reports (Black, 1993; Girder, 1996; Meltzoff, 1998; Schiavetti & Metz, 1997). Some of the guidelines that have been developed for reviewing published reports

Table 6.1

Factors To Consider in Assessing the Quality of Published Reports

Readership of a report, that is, the number and percentage of those who receive the publication and choose to read a report and then assign a value to it.

Letters to the editor of the publication commenting on the report.

Attention given to the report by the media.

Frequency and rapidity of citation of the report in references of other reports.

Republication or abstraction of the report in other professional journals and literature.

Perceived prestige of the journal in which the report appears.

Selection of the author by recognized authorities as meriting awards or identification as a "landmark article."

Selection of report for discussion in journal clubs.

Requests for permission to reprint or republish the report.

Quotation or citation of the paper in lectures by other professionals.

Formal or informal peer review of the paper after publication.

Note. Adapted from "The Quality of a Medical Article," by G. D. Lundburg and E. Williams, 1991, *Journal of American Medical Association, 265*(9), pp. 1161–1162.

are listed in Table 6.2. Perhaps the most important question for a critical reader to ask is "What does it mean?" (Isaac & Michael, 1987, p. 219). Polit and Hungler (1991) offered several different guidelines for evaluating published report, including (a) general guidelines to consider in conducting a written research critique; (b) research literature review; (c) theoretical/conceptual frameworks; (d) research hypotheses; (e) research designs; (f) sample plans; (g) self-reports such as interviews, questionnaires, and scales; (h) observational methods; (i) biophysiologic measures; (j) types of measurements; (k) quantitative analysis; (l) qualitative analysis; (m) interpretative dimension; (n) ethical aspects; and (o) presentation.

Many of the guidelines for reviewing published reports have been developed by professionals other than speech–language pathologists and audiologists. This may in part explain differences in strategies for evaluating reports. For example, in Table 6.2 one of the factors considered in assessing the quality of a medical report is "attention given to the report by the public media" (Lundberg & Williams, 1991). Media attention is usually not a factor in speech–language pathology and audiology. If there is media attention, it is often directed toward less-than-mainstream treatments and claims. For example, facilitated communication, fast forward, and auditory integration training have received media attention.

In reviewing the literature, attention should be given to unanswered questions and methodological strengths and weaknesses (Cone, 1993). A list of questions for the reader to ask when reading a report can help develop a systematic approach

that speeds up the process of critically reading published reports. Readers may use a checklist to read reports on their own or as part of a journal club and compare their findings with others (Riegelman & Hirsch, 1989). This series of questions could also be reconsidered by the same reader at a later time and compared with the first responses. That would assist readers in determining their consistency in critically reading published reports. Figure 6.1 is a checklist for evaluating various aspects of a research report as adequate or inadequate. Classifying observations into categories such as adequate or inadequate is the simplest strategy. Another evaluation strategy is to rank various items from poor to excellent, such as Schiavetti and Metz's (1997) guidelines for critical evaluation of research reports. This is a challenging task, even for an experienced journal reader.

For reviewing reports, Hyman (1995) suggested a rough ordinal scale from least to most valuable: (a) simply showing that the report is wrong; (b) showing not only that the report is wrong, but also what is right; (c) acknowledging the good points in the report; (d) allowing for the possibility the author might be wrong for good reason; and (e) showing that the report, if wrong, contributes new insights and integration to the topic under discussion.

The most comprehensive tool for the critical reader is *Evaluating Research in Communicative Disorders* by Schiavetti and Metz (1997). The book includes examples of critical reviews: one for speech disorders, one for language disorders, and one for audiology. Another comprehension tool is Black's (1993) Profiling Sheet, which provides specific criteria for var-

Table 6.2
Guidelines for Evaluating Published Reports

Reference	Description
American Psychological Association (1994)	Questions for evaluating quality of presentation Figure checklist Table checklist Manuscript checklist
Bailar and Mosteller (1988)	Guidelines for statistical reporting
Black (1993)	Profiling sheet
Braddom (1990)	54-item outline for writing and evaluating research papers
Cho and Bero (1994)	Methodologic Quality instrument
Cone (1993)	Guidelines for evaluating empirical studies
Coury (1991)	Three questions for reviewing articles
DePoy and Gitlin (1994)	Questions for analysis of research
Doehring (1988)	Narrative on how to read and evaluate research reports
Findley (1991)	Conceptual review of the literature
Fink (1998)	Checklist for conducting literature reviews
Gardner, Mechin, and Campbell (1986)	Checklist for assessing statistical content
Hegde (1994)	Outline for summary evaluation of research reports
Isaac and Michael (1987)	Form for the evaluation of an article Criteria for evaluation of a research report, article, or thesis
Justice et al. (1994)	18 fine-point ordinal questions for evaluating manuscript quality
Lundberg and Williams (1991)	11 criteria for determining the quality of an article
Maxwell and Satake (1997)	Research article questionnaire
Meltzoff (1998)	21-item checklist
Polit and Hungler (1991)	11 criteria for determining the quality of an article
Portney and Watkins (1993)	42-item questionnaire
Schiavetti and Metz (1997)	48-item checklist
Silverman (1993)	Evaluation checklist for validity, reliability, and generality

ious parameters considered in evaluating a report, including question/hypothesis, representatives, data quality, descriptive statistics, and inferential statistical analysis.

Internet

In recent years, concern has grown about the reliability of information on the Internet (Funk, 1998). S. D. McLeod (1998) is concerned "that a substantial proportion of clinical information on the Internet might be inaccurate, erroneous, misleading, or fraudulent." (p. 1663). Eysenbach and Diepsen (1998) believe "The quality of information on the Internet is extremely variable, limiting its use as a serious information source" (p. 1496).

Given the uneven quality of information on the Internet, it should be carefully evaluated. Criteria for evaluation of information on the Internet have been developed (Eysenbach & Diepsen, 1998; Tate & Alexander, 1996; Vicca, 1994).

Common Deficiencies

Knowing the common deficiencies in published reports may help readers recognize them more easily as they interpret reports. These deficiencies include problems in methodology, inadequate control of variables, inaccurate references and quotations, overgeneralization of the data, poor conceptualization of problem or approach, poor literature review, research design problems, statistical errors, and writing flaws such as uneven flow of content, very lengthy paragraphs, awkwardly worded sentences, and even incomplete sentences (R. J. Coelho & Saunders, 1997; Culatta, 1984; Thomas & Lawrence, 1990).

Training

It is important to learn critical reading. Students often have difficulty in making the transition between the type of reading required in most classes and the reading required for profes-

Checklist for Evaluating a Research Report

	Adequate	Inadequate
Significance of the problem investigated	☐	☐
Introduction and literature review		
Clear and complete	☐	☐
Objective, impartial, appropriately critical	☐	☐
Provided purpose for the present study	☐	☐
Statement of the problem		
Clear, replicable	☐	☐
Clear hypothesis or research questions	☐	☐
Methods		
Clear, adequate, replicable	☐	☐
Subject selection, treatment clear and appropriate	☐	☐
Research design readily understood	☐	☐
Adequate sample for data collection	☐	☐
Research design appropriate and correctly implemented	☐	☐
Results		
Stated unambiguously, objectively	☐	☐
Appropriate method of data analysis	☐	☐
Appropriate use of statistical procedures	☐	☐
Figures and tables used effectively	☐	☐
Data presentation orderly/logical	☐	☐
Interpreted appropriately	☐	☐
Discussion		
Results discussed adequately	☐	☐
Hypothesis rejected appropriately	☐	☐
Findings related to previous research	☐	☐
Implications of the study included	☐	☐
Suggestions included for additional research	☐	☐
Limitations of study discussed	☐	☐
References		
Included only works cited in text	☐	☐
Accurate and correct format	☐	☐
Appendix		
Necessary to understanding of report	☐	☐
Appropriate or suffient in length	☐	☐

Comments: _____

_____

Figure 6.1. Checklist for evaluating aspects of a research report as adequate or inadequate. *Note.* Adapted from *Clinical Research in Communication Disorders: Principles and Strategies*, by M. N. Hegde, 1994, Austin, TX: PRO-ED. Adapted with permission.

sional practice. Several reasons explain this difficulty: (a) limited previous knowledge and experience, (b) poor attitude, and (c) lack of training in critically reviewing published reports. Too often instructors will assign reviews of reports without providing guidance on how to approach the assignment. The result is often a trial-and-error approach to reading reports (Sorrell & Brown, 1991). Many students have had limited experience; they may have completed graduate training programs in speech–language pathology and audiology having read or written few, if any, critical reviews. Developing more capable critical readers should be an integral part of training in speech–language pathology and audiology.

Some students have been told or have convinced themselves that they cannot critically read published reports in communication disorders. Students should be made aware of the potential benefits to be gained from critically reading reports. Instructors' notations on reviews often emphasize the negative, ignore the positive features, and provide little guidance for revision. To be effective, faculty should communicate to students those strategies that facilitate critical reading. Unfortunately, many practicing speech–language pathologists and audiologists learn to critically read the literature the same way students do, by trial and error. Speech–language pathologists and audiologists should not hesitate to make judgments about published reports and compare them with those of others who are more knowledgeable (Hegde, 1994).

Students need written guidelines to critically review published reports. These guidelines should include detailed information about the purposes and expectations of an assigned review and criteria to be used when reading. Providing examples of reviews as well as published reports may be helpful. Another approach to learning is teaching what one thinks he or she knows about a report to someone else. Locke, Silverman, and Spindoso (1998) believe this is the best way to learn how to critically evaluate a published report. Examples of reviews to illustrate the process of evaluation of weaknesses and strengths were provided by Schiavetti and Metz (1997). Additional examples of reviews can be found in Girder's (1996) *Evaluating Research Articles* and Meltzoff's (1998) *Critical Thinking About Research,* which include a variety of studies.

Journal Group

Another approach to learning how to critically read published reports is participating in a journal group, which meets periodically to review and discuss journal reports. Members of the group are responsible for critically reviewing selected reports, comparing their reviews, and discussing application of the information to clinical practice.

Markert (1989) described a monthly journal club to teach essential components of research design, research methods, and statistics in a manner applicable to clinical practice. Journal clubs help professionals learn to be lifelong critical readers of the professional literature. To establish a framework, the first meeting is devoted to reports that discuss research designs and common statistical methods used in journals. Subsequently, each month, one of the journal club members volunteers to select and discuss a report. Two weeks before a meeting each member of the group is given a copy of the report to be discussed, a guide for presenting the report to the group, and a list of related questions to facilitate critical review of the report. The guide for presenting the report is a checklist in question form about the elements of the report: the purpose, design, methods, results, and conclusions. Some of the stimulus questions are general and others are specific to the report and help members determine the quality of the report, the appropriateness of the data and method, and the validity of the conclusions. Fagan (n.d.) and ASHA (1998b) provide detailed descriptions of journal clubs, including advice on forming a journal club, reading for group discussions, and determining the moderator's role. This information is presented in Table 6.3.

An important benefit of journal clubs for speech–language pathologists and audiologists is that they provide a way of earning continuing education (CE) units from the American Speech-Language-Hearing Association (ASHA). The CE division of ASHA should be contacted before a journal club is organized or shortly thereafter.

Reviews of the Literature

Another resource for learning to critically review reports is work that reviews a specific topic or issue. Such reviews have been published about a variety of topics in communication disorders such as dysarthria (Yorkston, 1996), voice quality (R. D. Kent, 1996), language impairment (Coelho, DeRuyter, & Stein, 1996; Harris, 1996; Holland, Davida, DeRuyter & Stein, 1996), articulation and phonological disorders (Gierut, 1998), hearing loss (Carney & Moeller, 1998; Weinstein, 1996), preschool language tests (Plante & Vance, 1994; Sturner et al., 1994), stuttering (Conture, 1996), and voice disorders (Ramig & Verdolini, 1998). Additional sources include reviews in *Asha* and letters to the editor published in ASHA journals. Letters to the editor are analyses and commentaries by readers of reports. They often focus on methodological problems in a report or provide alternate interpretations of the data (Maxwell & Satake, 1997).

Impact on Clinical Practice

For clinical speech–language pathology or audiology, the main test of a report's importance is the extent to which it modifies clinical practice. Methods of assessing the impact of a report on clinical practice have received little attention and no indicators are available.

The *Journal of the American Medical Association* published a series of articles about using articles to make clinical deci-

Table 6.3
Journal Clubs

Advantages

Know latest developments in field

Enhance learning

Increase reading retention and comprehension through group discussions and interaction

Discover new ways to apply learning to clinical practice

Earn continuing education credits in flexible manner

Translate research into clinical practice

Participate actively in the learning process

Group Formation and Purpose

Limit number of members to at least three and no more than 10.

Determine group direction: general or specific focus.

Reading for Group Discussion

Advance preparation is essential.

Why did the author write the report? What did the author intend for you to learn or do from reading and studying the report?

What are the various concepts or positions expressed in the report? Are the conclusions justified by the data?

How does the information presented in the report relate to your current understanding and knowledge in the area? Did it add something, reaffirm, cast doubt, contradict?

How do you apply what was learned in the report to clinical practice? What could you do differently in your practice given this new knowledge? How will this change your practice?

Does this report suggest other things to investigate on the topic? How can you get more information? (further readings including other reports referred to in the reference section, conferences, discussions with colleagues, bibliographies)

Moderator

Facilitates the group's learning and keeps the discussion on track.

Introduces the topic for discussion, keeps the discussion on topic, and summarizes at the end of the discussion.

Prepares questions in advance of the meeting to provoke discussion when needed.

Maintains a nonthreatening atmosphere, encourages members to participate, keeps one member from dominating the discussion.

Avoids giving an initial summary presentation of the report to the group. Assumes everyone is prepared to take an active part in a group discussion of the article.

Ensures that the group adheres to its schedule.

Note. Adapted from Fagan (n.d.) and American Speech-Language-Hearing Association (1998b).

sions (Guyatt et al., 1997; Guyatt, Sackett, & Cook, 1994; Laupacis, Wells, Richardson, & Tuswell, 1994; Wilson, Hayward, Tunis, Bass, & Guyatt, 1996). This framework could be used by speech–language pathologists and audiologists to assess reports and decide whether the information will benefit their clients. Information is organized to answer three questions:

1. Are the results of the report valid?

2. What are the results?

3. Will the results help in treating clients?

Reading Clinical Research Reports: Summary

Sources for strategies that a reader can take to critically review published reports have been the major focus of this section. The suggestions are summarized as follows: (a) use published guidelines; (b) be aware of common deficiencies; (c) understand factors important to the quality of a report; (d) obtain training; (e) practice reviewing reports; (f) obtain examples of critical reviews; (g) be a member of a journal group; (h) compare reviews with those of other readers; (i) read and assess review articles; (j) read letters to the editor; and (k) consider the impact of a report on clinical practice. Critical reading of published reports can facilitate appropriate interpretation and utilization of research findings. Further information about issues related to critically reviewing reports in speech–language pathology and audiology is needed. This includes but is not limited to (a) when and how speech–language pathologists and audiologists learn to critically review reports; (b) what the most effective strategies for reviewing reports are; (c) what the impact of critically reading reports on clinical practice is; (d) how speech–language pathologists and audiologists use published reports to make clinical decisions; and (e) how critical analysis of reports be can recognized for continuing education credits.

Writing Clinical Research Reports

Clinical research is a process that starts with the clinical situation, leads to formulating and answering the questions, is followed by dissemination of the findings, and eventually results in its integration into clinical practice (Findley, 1989). It is a mistake to separate research and clinical practice (Apel, 1999; Connell & McReynolds, 1988; Cornett & Chabon, 1988; Cox & West, 1986; Doehring, 1988; Hegde, 1994). Hamre (1972), Kamhi (1984, 1995), and Ringel (1972) identified similar activities in research and clinical practice. Both clinicians and researchers (a) identify and analyze problems; (b) develop and implement procedures; (c) collect, analyze, and interpret data; (d) make decisions on data; (e) maintain data records; (f) report findings; and (g) conduct activities within professional and ethical guidelines. Research should be an integral part of the clinical service delivery process. Ongoing research is necessary to study clinical service delivery and to ensure quality services to consumers. Findley (1989) described several additional reasons for doing clinical research: (a) facilitating the objective, rather than subjective, recording of daily notes; (b) motivating clinicians and forestalling burnout when client improvement is not evident; (c) allowing reasoned choice among intervention options; (d) producing accountable, responsible clinicians; (e) maintaining and expanding programs by being effective and efficient; (f) enabling staff to develop professionally and not become stagnant technicians; (g) adding credibility to the profession; (h) developing an understanding of some basic process of conducting research; and (i) building upon previous research. Research is also reported for other reasons, which are listed in Table 6.4.

Unfortunately, speech–language pathologists and audiologists often perpetuate the traditional fallacy that they can be either clinicians or researchers, but not both. For the most part, clinicians have not made research an integral part of their clinical practice. Clinicians often feel they do not have time to do research. Those clinicians who do research often simply make

time. Silverman (1993) indicated that research need not be particularly time consuming. Other reasons why research is not reported are listed in Table 6.5.

Time-management strategies as well as type of research design might facilitate research productivity (Boice, 1989; Connell & Thompson, 1986; Henson, 1999; Silverman, 1993). Single-subject research designs require less time because clinicians who know this approach can collect data while providing clinical services. Use of single-subject designs can provide answers to many clinically relevant questions. Connell and McReynolds (1988) indicated that "individual contact with a client over an extended time interval is the requirement for implementation of single-subject experimental designs" (p. 1062). Chart reviews and clinical data can be used for exploratory or retrospective studies (Findley & Daum, 1989). Clinical research is complete only when the findings are reported in a written report or oral presentation. This is the final step in the research process. If research findings are not formally reported, their impact will be limited (American Psychological Association, 1994; Chial, 1985; Silverman, 1993).

In this section, eight areas of writing clinical research reports are discussed: (a) formats for disseminating clinical research, (b) authorship, (c) types of written reports, (d) preparation and organization of clinical research reports, (e) where to submit clinical research reports, (f) writing style, (g) word processors, and (h) ethical issues in reporting clinical research.

Formats for Disseminating Clinical Research

Written reports and oral presentations are the two main formats for disseminating research (Silverman, 1993). Written reports are the most frequently used format and typically are published as chapters in books or as articles in professional journals. Oral presentations typically consist of talks, poster sessions, or exhibits at local, state, national, or international professional meetings. Poster sessions have become a widespread feature of professional meetings (Beal, Lynch, & Moore, 1989; Bordens & Abbott, 1988; Cooper, Hersch, & Trapp, 1988; Simmonds, 1984). The poster is a display of research material on a vertical panel and usually requires the presence of the author to discuss the work. Poster sessions allow attendees to select the information they wish to receive, and to receive considerable information in a short period of time. Other formats for disseminating research include audiotapes, computer software programs, videotapes, and motion picture films.

Assigning Authorship

Co-authorship and collaboration are commonplace (Kirsch, 1995). An individual's approval must be obtained before that person can be listed as an author (O'Connor & Woodford, 1977). Any individual making a major contribution to a

Table 6.4
Reasons Research Is Reported

Reason	References
"Can do/will do" attitude; professional recognition	Kirby, 1989
Opportunity to be creative	Drew & Hardman, 1985
Employment policy: promotion, tenure, merit	Hegde, 1994; Higdon & Friel-Patti, 1987
Clarification, explanation, and organization of ideas	American Psychological Association, 1994; Hegde, 1994
Professional reputation; individual and institutional productivity	Higdon & Friel-Patti, 1987
Satisfying curiosity	Findley & Daum, 1989; Hegde, 1994
Enhancing continuing education and professional growth	American Psychological Association, 1994; Chial, 1985; Drew & Hardman, 1985
Clinical service mandates experimentation	Perkins, 1985
Application of computer technology	R. D. Kent & Fair, 1985
Solving problems	Hegde, 1994
"Solving the ills of society"	Drew & Hardman, 1985, p. 6
"Just plain fun"	Drew & Hardman, 1985, p. 6; Kirby, 1989
Research team	Grabois & Fuhrer, 1988
Administrative support	R. Kent, 1983
Facilitates networking	Ludlow, 1986
Scholarly obligation	Hunter & Kuh, 1987

research report should be listed as an author. Authorship includes not only those who do the actual writing but also those who have made other substantial contributions to the research (American Psychological Association, 1994). According to the American Psychological Association (1994), substantial professional contributions include "formulating the problem or hypothesis, structuring the experimental design, organizing and conducting the statistical analysis, interpreting the results, or writing a major portion of the paper" (p. 294). Not to be included as authors are individuals who simply advise or provide technical assistance in the usual course of their work. One's department head or other senior colleagues should not be listed automatically unless they made significant contributions to the research.

The order of authorship should be determined in relation to the degree of contribution (Drew & Hardman, 1985). The individual making the greatest contribution should be senior author; the others are listed in order of their relative contributions. If the contribution is relatively equal, order can be determined alphabetically, by a flip of the coin, or by some other method that is mutually acceptable. Members of research teams often take turns at being named as first author. Lesser contributions may be credited in an acknowledgment.

Types of Written Reports

Written reports are published in a variety of professional journals, including those of ASHA, state speech–language–hearing associations, and educational and health care associations. Familiarity with journals is the best way to determine how appropriate a research report is for a specific journal (Fuchs & Fuchs, 1993). Published reports range in length from less than a page to more than 100 pages; most are between 6 and 12 pages (Silverman, 1993). Accepted papers may be published as articles, reports, clinical exchanges, case reports, or letters to the editor.

Journals that classify papers as articles or reports usually do so on the basis of length; longer papers are classified as

Table 6.5
Reasons Research Is Not Reported

Reason	References
Too frivolous and too much like the "ivory tower"	Drew & Hardman, 1985
Nonsupportive administration	Chial, 1985
Unfavorable institutional settings	R. Kent, 1983; R. D. Kent & Fair, 1985
Lack of support network consisting of colleagues, staff, technicians, friends, and scholars at other locations	Chial, 1985; Grabois & Fuhrer, 1988; Ventry & Schiavetti, 1986
Attitudes such as bewilderment, uncertainty, impatience, boredom, frustration, and defeatism	American Psychological Association, 1994; Chial, 1985
Routine drudgery	Kerlinger, 1973; Shearer, 1982
Fear of rejection and/or criticism	Culatta, 1984; Shearer, 1982
Time-consuming	Chial, 1985; Henson, 1999
Halo effect: Most of my colleagues don't publish	Henson, 1999; Perkins, 1985
Limited research training	R. Kent, 1983; R. D. Kent & Fair, 1985; Shearer, 1982
Lack of confidence	R. Kent, 1983; R. D. Kent & Fair, 1985
Lack of rewards	R. Kent, 1983; R. D. Kent & Fair, 1985
Lack of time	R. Kent, 1983; R. D. Kent & Fair, 1985; Laney, 1982
Job definition and expectations	R. Kent, 1983
Disappointment in results	Shearer, 1982
Disenchantment with the topic	Shearer, 1982
Writer's block	Mack & Skjei, 1979

articles (Silverman, 1993). The type of research reported also may be a consideration. Papers that are philosophical or conceptual, or that synthesize research, are classified as articles, whereas those that are data-based, descriptive, or experimental studies are classified as reports. Organization is the same for both types of papers.

Clinical exchange reports are relatively short reports about clinically relevant issues. Case reports or studies are descriptions of individuals who are noteworthy for some reason. Such reports contain a single case study or several related case studies.

Letters to the editor often are critical responses to recently published papers in the same journal. They also may be statements of points of view, brief summaries of pilot work, or clinical case studies.

Preparation and Organization of Clinical Research Reports

Steps in publishing a paper are listed in Table 6.6. Many of these steps apply with suitable modification to oral presentations.

Before preparing a report, it is helpful to review published reports for organization and style. Another way to learn how to prepare reports is to consult references about writing. Several sources for guidelines are listed in Table 6.7.

The most relevant guide to review when preparing a written report to submit for publication is the most recent "information for authors" issued by the journal to which you plan to submit (O'Connor & Woodford, 1977; Silverman, 1993). Some journals publish this information in every issue; others

Table 6.6
Steps in Publishing a Paper in a Journal

1. Assess your work; decide what, when, and where to publish.

2. Obtain and review the instructions to authors of the journal chosen.

3. Decide authorship.

4. Draft a working title and abstract.

5. Decide on the basic form of the paper.

6. Collect the material under the major headings chosen.

7. Design tables, including titles and footnotes; design or select figures and illustrations, including titles and legends.

8. Obtain permission to reproduce any previously published material.

9. Write a topic outline and, possibly, a sentence outline.

10. Write or dictate a preliminary draft of the text.

11. Check accuracy of the references assembled.

12. Put away the manuscript for a few days.

13. Review the paper.

14. Check the tables, figures, and illustrations; make the final revisions.

15. Reread the references cited and check their accuracy. Check for consistency. Reduce the number of abbreviations and footnotes.

16. Retype the paper (first draft).

17. Correct the grammar and refine the style.

18. Make several copies of the corrected paper (second draft).

19. Ask for comments from co-authors and colleagues.

20. Make any necessary alterations.

21. Compose a new title and abstract suitable for information retrieval. List the index terms. Assemble the manuscript.

22. Compile the reference list, cross-check references against the text, and ensure that all biographical details are correct.

23. Retype manuscript (third draft). Proofread it.

24. Obtain a final critical review from a senior colleague.

25. Make any final corrections (final draft).

26. Write a cover letter to the editor, enclosing copies of letters giving permission to reproduce any previously published material or to cite unpublished work.

27. Check that all parts of the paper are present, and submit as many copies as specified to the editor.

28. Editor acknowledges receipt of manuscript.

29. Editor reviews manuscript.

30. Acceptance; Acceptance conditional on satisfactory revision; Rejection encouraging revision; Rejection; Celebrate; Submit revised manuscript to editor; Revise, resubmit manuscript.

31. Complete copyright transfer form; return it to editor.

32. Review edited manuscript, answer questions asked by reviewers, and return to editor.

33. Editor sends manuscript to typesetter for typesetting.

34. Editor sends manuscript, proofs, and reprint order form to author.

35. Proofread and return proofs and manuscript within specified time.

36. Journal is printed and released.

Table 6.7
Guides for Writing

Author	Year	Title
American Speech-Language-Hearing Association	1991–1992	*The Publication Process: A Guide for Authors*
American Psychological Association	1994	*Publication Manual of the American Psychological Association*
Burnard	1992	*Writing for Health Professionals: A Manual for Writers*
Dalton & Dalton	1990	*The Student's Guide to Good Writing*
Davis	1997	*Scientific Papers and Presentations*
Day	1994	*How To Write and Publish a Scientific Paper*
Hegde	1991	*Singular Manual of Textbook Preparation*
Hegde	1998	*A Book on Scientific and Professional Writing for Speech–Language Pathology*
Huth	1990	*How To Write and Publish Papers in the Medical Sciences*
Strunk & White	1999	*The Elements of Style*
Szuchman	1999	*Writing with Style: APA Style Made Easy*

publish it at regular intervals (e.g., in one issue a year); and others provide the information only on request.

The organization for written reports and oral presentations is essentially the same. The two ways in which oral reports differ from written reports are in style and length. Oral reports are usually less formal and more redundant than written reports. Also, oral reports are less detailed because of time limitations (Silverman, 1993). Research reports usually have most, if not all, of the following parts: (a) title, (b) abstract or summary, (c) introduction, (d) methodology, (e) results, (f) discussion, (g) acknowledgments, (h) references, and (i) appendixes. The purpose and content of each section have been described by the American Psychological Association (1994), Forscher and Wertz (1970), Hegde (1994), Kerlinger (1973), O'Connor and Woodford (1977), Shearer (1982), and Silverman (1993).

In recent years, several journals have adopted a format for more informative or structured abstracts. Information contained in these abstracts for original studies and literature reviews is presented in Table 6.8. More informative abstracts can facilitate peer review before publication, assist readers in finding reports that are scientifically sound and applicable to their clinical practice, and permit more precise computerized literature searches (R. B. Haynes et al., 1996).

Where To Submit Clinical Research Reports

The final task in the research process is disseminating the findings. This usually involves locating a professional meeting at which to submit an oral report, locating a journal in which to submit a written report, or both, since many papers presented at professional meetings are later published. Figure 6.2 is a checklist that writers should consider before submitting a manuscript for publication. The outlets most often used by speech–language pathologists and audiologists for dissemination of research findings are convention programs and publications of state speech–language pathology or audiology associations (Silverman, 1993).

Writing Style

Research reports should be accurate and concise. Vocabulary should be appropriate. "Academispeak" or the jargon and gibberish of academia that is used by academics and self-important students to elevate "prestige" should be avoided (Friske, 1990, p. 26). Reading published research reports can be helpful, as well as consulting references about writing research reports including American Psychological Association (1994), Fowler (1980), Gibaldi and Achtert (1984), O'Connor and Woodford (1977), and Strunk and White (1999). Most books on research methods provide information about writing research reports (Bordens & Abbott, 1988; Hegde, 1994; Polit & Hungler, 1991).

Sexist language should be avoided. ASHA (1993) does not condone communication that intentionally or unintentionally uses biased or discriminatory gender terms. It is inherently discriminatory language, either spoken or written, that implies an unjustified sexual bias against an individual or a group, usually women but sometimes men (Schneider & Soto, 1989). Because of the increased awareness that language can perpetuate stereotypes, sexist language should be avoided by speakers and writers (Gefuert, 1985; Kidder & Judd, 1986). Cheney (1983) believes that, because "women are equal partners with men" (p. 187), nothing is more pathetic than a writer out of touch with the realities of time. One of the most misused personal pronouns is *he*. It is frequently used to refer to someone of unidentified sex, such as a child, client, customer, or student (Hegde, 1994; Troyka, 1990). Indiscriminate use of personal pronouns may imply that all authors, bankers, department heads, doctors, editors, executives, firefighters, lawyers, police officers, presidents, or professors are male. An often inappropriately used noun that implies sexism is *man* (e.g., chair*man* of an academic department or organization; in such case, *chairperson* or *chair* is appropriate).

In 1979, the ASHA Committee on Equality of Sexes adopted the American Psychological Association's *Guidelines for Nonsexist Language* (ASHA, 1979). More recently, ASHA (1993) published guidelines for gender equality in language use. These guidelines provide specific suggestions and examples for avoiding sexist language. Other useful references are available, such as *The Handbook of Nonsexist Writing* by C. Miller and Swift (1988), *Nonsexist Communicator* by Sorrels (1983), and *The Elements of Nonsexist Usage* by Dumond (1990).

"Person first" language should be used. As a result of the Individuals with Disabilities Education Act of 1990, all references to disabilities should be written with the individual placed first (Stein & Cutler, 1996). ASHA encourages contributors to use person-first language in writing manuscripts. For example, *adult with aphasia* is correct, whereas *the aphasic adult* is incorrect. Several years earlier Knepflar (1976) indicated the need to "refrain from labeling people by the names of their problems . . . emphasizing the fact that primarily they are people, and secondarily they have a problem" (p. 45).

Word Processing

A word processor is invaluable in preparing reports by those familiar with and comfortable using word processing (Doehring, 1988; Luey, 1987; Mulkerne & Mulkerne, 1988). Every aspect of writing is facilitated with word processing software. Specific sections of a report can be kept in separate files. References can be added and deleted as needed. Special programs are available for graphics. Revisions are easily made (Doehring, 1988) (see Chapter 5).

Table 6.8
Information Needed for More Informative Abstracts

Original Articles

1. Objective: exact questions addressed by the article

2. Design: the basic design of the study

3. Setting: the location and level of clinical care

4. Patients or participants: the manner of selection and number of patients or participants who entered and completed the study

5. Interventions: the exact treatment or intervention, if any

6. Main outcome measures: the primary study outcome measure as planned before data collection began

7. Results: the key findings

8. Conclusions: key conclusions including direct clinical applications

Review Articles

1. Purpose: the primary objective of the review article

2. Data sources: a succinct summary of data sources

3. Study selection: the number of studies selected for review and how they were selected

4. Data extraction: rules for abstracting data and how they were applied

5. Results of data synthesis: the method of data synthesis and key results

6. Conclusions: key conclusions, including potential applications and research needs

Note. Adapted from "More Informative Abstracts Revisited," by R. B. Haynes, C. D. Mulrow, E. J. Huth, D. G. Altman, and M. J. Gardner, 1996, *Cleft Palate–Craniofacial Journal, 13*(1).

Checklist for Submitting a Manuscript

General

☐ Type entire manuscript double-spaced, with a ragged right margin, in a 12-point font.

☐ Supply running head (short title) limited to 50 characters.

☐ Type the full manuscript title on the first page of text, after the summary (formerly abstract).

☐ Eliminate boldface in headings. (See APA [American Psychological Association] Manual, p. 91, for heading styles.)

☐ Number all pages, except actual figures, in sequence, starting with the title page.

☐ Italicize letters used as statistical symbols/algebraic variables (e.g., t test of $p < .001$).

☐ Arrange manuscript parts in this order: title page, summary page, text, references, author note, appendixes, footnotes, tables, figure captions, figures.

☐ Put corresponding author's current postal and e-mail address in the author's note, on the title page. The title page should note institutional affiliation of all authors at the time the research report was done.

Text

☐ Use hard return to indicate new paragraphs: DO NOT use hard returns for line breaks.

☐ Cite multiple published works within parentheses alphabetically by first author's surname. When not within parentheses, order does not matter.

☐ Link last author's name in a multiple-author citation within parentheses to preceding author's name with an ampersand (&). Outside parentheses, use "and."

☐ Cite a reference with six or more authors by noting the first author's surname plus "et al."

☐ Cite as many authors' surnames in sequence as is necessary to distinguish one multiple-authors citation from another, then add "et al."

☐ Indicate phonetic characters by enclosing them within slashes //. If necessary, write character on hard copy.

☐ Eliminate any unnecessary abbreviations (i.e., those that are not explained).

☐ Do not use sexist language. Use person-first language unless the result is too cumbersome. (See ASHA 1979, 1993 guidelines.)

References Section

☐ Supply full reference for any work (and ONLY those works) cited in text.

☐ Order references alphabetically by authors' names.

☐ Verify that spelling of authors' names and dates agree with text citation.

☐ Indent first line of each reference. Type subsequent lines flush left.

☐ Note full titles of journals and their volume numbers and the titles of books.

☐ Follow APA Manual, pp. 204–206 for citing chapters from multiauthored books.

☐ Supply inclusive page numbers for all articles from journals or articles/chapters from books.

Quotations/Copyright

☐ Provide page numbers in text for all direct quotations.

☐ Obtain written permission to use previously published materials, and enclose copy of the permission.

Tables

☐ Double space entire table and title.

☐ Supply heading for all columns (including the first).

☐ Use tab key, NOT the space bar, to create columns.

☐ Align decimal points in columns.

☐ Remove vertical rules from tables.

☐ Add "table continued" at the bottom of the page of any table that exceeds a page in length, and repeat column headings on subsequent pages.

Figures

☐ Identify all figures on the back with manuscript name and figure number.

Figure 6.2. Checklist for submitting a manuscript. *Note.* From *Manuscript Checklist*, by American Speech-Language-Hearing Association, 1998c, Rockville, MD: Author. Copyright 1998 by *Asha*. Reprinted with permission.

Ethical Issues in Reporting Clinical Research

Hegde (1994) believes "dissemination of research findings is an ethical responsibility of researchers" (p. 442). The 1990 ASHA Code of Ethics indicated "individuals should strive to increase knowledge within the profession and share research with colleagues" (p. 92).

There also are ethical issues related to reporting research. One issue is related to multiple publication of the same article in different professional journals. It is not appropriate to submit the same article to two professional journals at the same time. Simultaneous submission of a manuscript to multiple journals could result in self-plagiarism. Although multiple submissions create problems, it is a frequent occurrence (Henson, 1999). ASHA has a written policy that states no manuscript that is under consideration elsewhere should be submitted. Another issue is related to accuracy of references and quotations. It is the writer's responsibility to verify references and quotations. Roland (1976) believes verifying references and quotations is something many writers fail to do, even those whose articles appear in the published literature (Boyce & Banning, 1979; DeLacey, Record, & Wade, 1985; Eichorn & Yankauer, 1987; Evans, Nadjari, & Burchell, 1990; Foreman & Kirchoff, 1987; Key & Roland, 1977). Other issues are related to authorship and involve who should be listed as authors and the order of authorship (Drew & Hardman, 1985). The ASHA Code of Ethics (1990) addresses this issue: "Individuals should assign credit to those who have contributed to the publication in proportion to their contribution" (p. 92). Authorship was discussed earlier in this chapter.

Student Research Reports: Term Papers, Theses, and Dissertations

Unfortunately, students do not get enough training and practice in writing research reports during graduate school (Van Wagenen, 1991). Student research reports include term papers, theses, and dissertations. The sequence of informational presentation is nearly always the same as that of other research reports (Shearer, 1982). Student research reports should be written in the American Psychological Association (APA) format (Doehring, 1988). Szuchman's (1999) book, *Writing with Style*, provides a method for students to learn to write APA-style research papers. Students should review their papers before submitting them to an instructor. See Figure 6.3 for a checklist to help avoid the most common errors in preparing a paper. Guides to writing papers including theses and doctoral dissertations are available elsewhere (Cone, 1993; Dalton & Dalton, 1990; Davis & Parker, 1979; Fitzpatrick, Secrist, & Wright, 1998; Madsen, 1992; Mulkerne & Mulkerne, 1988; Rudestam & Newton, 1992; Sternberg, 1981; Van Wagenen, 1991).

Students should consult their training programs, as well as their instructors, for specific regulations regarding the recommended style for research reports. Not all programs require the APA format used in ASHA journals. This is unfortunate because the student would be better prepared for postacademic writing by using ASHA's recommended style (Shearer, 1982).

Chial (1985) provides several suggestions for students about research. These suggestions include recognizing

- the role of interpersonal dynamics
- the role of intrapersonal dynamics
- that much of the research report is predetermined in format
- that success is more likely if the research design is simple and details are attended to
- the importance and limitations of technical tools
- that student research is a learning experience, and significant learning cannot occur in the absence of error
- that good writing demands hard work
- that the research experience will change a person as a scholar, as a professional, and perhaps even as an individual

Dalton and Dalton's (1990) guidelines to writing for students relate to

- developing topics
- seeking support
- taking risks
- being flexible
- treating writing as a game
- listening to advice and suggestions offered by peers and professors
- reading for both content and style
- writing at every opportunity
- staying committed
- avoiding boring traditional approaches

The organization and issues related to research reports are similar for term papers and other student reports. The primary way in which term papers and reports differ from research reports is the level of training of the authors. Term papers and reports are done during academic training. A second difference is the format for evaluation. Research reports are usually

Checklist for Students Preparing a Research Report

The questions listed below concern the most common oversights in paper preparation. Review these items carefully before submitting a paper to an instructor.

Yes	No	
☐	☐	Is the entire paper double spaced?
☐	☐	Is the paper clean and neatly prepared?
☐	☐	Are all pages numbered in the right-hand corner in sequence?
☐	☐	Is the title concise, accurate, and informative?
☐	☐	Is the title 12 to 15 words?
☐	☐	Is the abstract 100 to 175 words?
☐	☐	Is the introduction clear and complete?
☐	☐	Does the introduction section specifically state the purpose of the paper?
☐	☐	Are personal references minimized by not using words such as *I* and *we*?
☐	☐	Is sexist language avoided?
☐	☐	Is person-first language used?
☐	☐	Have unnecessary words and repetition been eliminated?
☐	☐	Is the use of tense (present, past, and/or future) consistent?
☐	☐	Is the paper free from grammatical errors?
☐	☐	Is each paragraph longer than a sentence, but not much longer than one typed page?
☐	☐	Are headings used effectively?
☐	☐	Has too much material been drawn from one source?
☐	☐	Does the paper accomplish the objectives as stated in the introduction?
☐	☐	Are the conclusions based on evidence presented in the paper?
☐	☐	Does the paper show scholarly effort?
☐	☐	Are tables and figures used to supplement the text?
☐	☐	Are suggestions for future research identified?
☐	☐	Are clinical implications stated?
☐	☐	Does the discussion summarize the current problems and limitations?
☐	☐	Does the discussion stick to the point and confine itself to what can be concluded from the findings?
☐	☐	Is the report clearly written and concise?
☐	☐	Is the report well organized?
☐	☐	Is there a current, thorough, and accurate review of the literature?
☐	☐	Are inclusive page numbers for all articles or book chapters listed in the references?
☐	☐	Are page numbers provided in the text for all quotations?
☐	☐	Do the references follow APA style?
☐	☐	Are references cited both in text and in the reference list?
☐	☐	Are the acknowledgments clear and concise?

Figure 6.3. Checklist for students preparing a research report.

peer reviewed, whereas term papers and reports are typically evaluated by a single instructor.

Writing Clinical Research Reports: Summary

For a variety of reasons, many audiologists and speech–language pathologists do not report research findings. This is regrettable for several reasons: (a) research is incomplete until the findings are disseminated in an oral report, a written report, or both; (b) the impact of research and scholarship is limited; (c) clinical management strategies cannot be effectively updated; and (d) when information is not shared with colleagues, a general failure to build upon the knowledge base of the profession results. Clinicians should be aware of factors that are counterproductive to reporting research. It is important that clinicians be critical reviewers of research in order to update clinical practice, and be sufficiently involved in the profession to willingly and steadfastly contribute to and report research.

 Discussion Questions

1. Why should research reports be critically reviewed?

2. How can research reports be critically reviewed?

3. What are the common deficiencies of research reports?

4. How can one learn to read critically?

5. Why is it difficult to read critically?

6. How is authorship determined?

7. What is "person first" language?

8. Explain the differences between theses and dissertations.

9. Why should speech–language pathology and audiology students be familiar with APA formats?

10. What factors should be considered in evaluating the quality of published reports?

11. How can the prestige of a journal be determined?

12. What is peer review? How does it affect authors and journals?

13. Describe the advantages and disadvantages of belonging to a journal club.

14. Why is research reported?

15. Why is research not reported?

Oral Reports

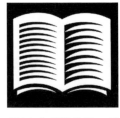

Speech–language pathologists and audiologists give oral reports throughout their professional careers. Whenever a diagnostic or treatment session takes place, the clinician should present an appropriate oral report to the client, the family, or other professionals. An oral report is any spoken factual statement requiring preparation and organization. Like the written report, the oral report should be clear, informative, and appropriate. Oral reports vary in style, length, complexity, and formality. Regardless of the level of formality, oral reports should communicate information that people will understand and use. Oral reports are used often because they are both time and cost efficient. An oral report may precede the written report or follow the written report to provide further information or opportunity for discussion and consultation (J. Farmer, 1989). Information about oral reports in speech–language pathology and audiology is limited. The purpose of this chapter is to discuss oral reports that are used in clinical situations.

Oral reports include informal reports and formal reports such as staffing and grand rounds. Both informal and formal oral reports require skill in listening as well as in speaking. S. Farmer (1989) described a number of strategies for developing competence in listening.

Informal Oral Reports

At the least formal level, the oral report may consist of a discussion with someone else. For example, following an evaluation, the clinician should meet with the family to discuss the evaluation results and to provide recommendations. During treatment, the clinician should meet with the family to obtain their suggestions and to discuss treatment plans and progress (Sanders, 1972). There also may be situations in which oral reports are used to supplement written reports. Telephone discussions may be helpful, but direct face-to-face discussion is much more likely to be effective (Knepflar, 1976).

Formal Oral Reports

Staffing and case presentations or grand rounds are a more formal type of oral report. Staffing may consist of making decisions after the speech–language–hearing evaluation or reviewing individual client treatment. It may also consist of a multidisciplinary team approach in which members of the team provide expertise in matters relevant to diagnosis and treatment of a disorder or disease, educational processes, or other matters (Nicolosi, Harryman, & Kresheck, 1989; Sanders, 1972).

Immediately after the speech–language–hearing evaluation and before the discussion with the family, the clinician or clinicians make certain decisions, such as these: Is there a speech, language, or hearing problem? If so, what is the problem, how severe is it, and what is the prognosis? What recommendations should be made? Eisenstadt (1972) reported that parents expressed discomfort about inadequate explanations of diagnostic findings, and inappropriate or vague levels of language used by clinicians. Later research indicates that clinicians have improved in this area. Shipley and McCroskey (1978) found that the majority of parents believe that diagnostic findings were adequately explained. More recently, Watson and Thompson (1983) reported that nearly all parents (90% to 93%) indicated that they understood diagnostic information in conferences and written reports.

The importance of repetition in providing information to clients and their families should be considered. Clinicians often forget that they have spent considerable time developing their understanding of communication disorders; however, they often expect the family to understand in one hurried session.

According to Cornett and Chabon (1988), "all clients should be staffed as part of a clinician's commitment to the process of continuity of care and to the assessment of the quality of care" (p. 108). Staffing of individual clients, sometimes referred to as case reports, case presentations, or case conferences, involves reporting and organizing client information and reviewing diagnostic reports and treatment plans. A staffing report should be concise. In most situations it should last no longer than 3 minutes (R. Miller & Groher, 1990).

Thus, the clinician should concentrate on only the most relevant information. Staffing provides an opportunity for different clinicians to give their views about a client. It allows clinicians to learn from other clinicians; thus it also serves as a continuing educational medium.

A staffing summary outline helps in preparing for staffing (see Table 7.1). This summary usually includes a report about

Table 7.1

Staffing Summary of Information Outline

I. Introduction
    A. First name of client
    B. Age
    C. Number of semesters in treatment

II. Reasons for staffing/specific questions

III. Significant History
    A. Medical
    B. Developmental
    C. Social
        1. Family constellation
        2. School
        3. Traumatic experiences
        4. Socioeconomic level
        5. Parental/spouse involvement in remediation
    D. Other agencies seen/services received

IV. Speech and Language Services
    A. Initial diagnosis
        1. Reasons for referral
        2. Recommendations
    B. General statement regarding goals and progress of previous treatment
    C. Present Treatment
        1. Goals
        2. Procedures
        3. Progress
        4. Samples (either audiotape or videotape)
    D. Family education

V. Behavioral Observations
    A. Home
    B. School
    C. Treatment

the relevant case history data, diagnostic information, date treatment was initiated, cumulative number of sessions, specific treatment methods used, progress observed, and future plans and recommendations. Client staffings may be facilitated by using videotapes or audiotapes of clients; inviting consultants or other professionals who are directly involved with the client to attend and participate in staffing; and allowing time for discussion and questions (Cornett & Chabon, 1988). It is helpful to have guidelines in preparing for and reviewing a staffing. See Figure 7.1 for a checklist for evaluation of staffing. A report of the staffing should be filed in the client's master file (see Figure 7.2).

The standards for accreditation by ASHA's (1995a) Professional Services Board require evidence of program evaluation and quality assurance including formal evaluation of individual client treatment. The evaluation system must be documented. This includes conferences held with other clin-

icians to review client progress, to develop further treatment plans, and to maintain an integrated and coordinated program.

Multidisciplinary team staffing provides an opportunity to integrate the information gathered during the different professional evaluations so that it can be shared with the family and the referral sources (Holm & McCartin, 1978). Many teams refer to this process as a staffing or case conference. This process provides an opportunity for all the different professionals to give their views about a client and serves to maximize information and effort (Spriestersbach, 1968). Most teams include local professionals who are involved with the client. Some teams, as a rule or an option, include the family in this decision-making conference (Dorenberg, 1976).

Conflicting views should be considered and controversies resolved. How this is done varies; often the same team goes about this task differently at different times. There are, however, some general principles that apply to all team staffings. The professional in charge of staffing should be the case manager. This individual should plan the staffing in advance. The emphasis of a staffing should be an exchange of information. The best way to ensure this is to follow some basic do's and don'ts (see Figure 7.3).

Responsibility for a productive staffing is usually that of the person in charge, but there are rules for the participants. The most important rule is to speak up—important information

---

Staffing Checklist

Yes	No	
☐	☐	1. Was the reason for staffing clear?
☐	☐	2. Was the clinician knowledgeable about the client?
☐	☐	3. Was relevant history information presented?
☐	☐	4. Were diagnosis and/or treatment of speech–language–hearing problems adequately described?
☐	☐	5. Did the clinician answer questions effectively and efficiently?
☐	☐	6. Was the presentation organized, unified, coherent, and logical?
☐	☐	7. Was the vocabulary appropriate for those attending the staffing?
☐	☐	8. Were the recommendations for treatment appropriate?
☐	☐	9. Was audiovisual material used to supplement the oral presentation?

Figure 7.1. Staffing checklist.

should never be withheld. If participants disagree with what goes on, they should say so. The professional approach is to attempt to resolve disagreements and problems.

Case reports or presentations may be used to teach students spoken and written language skills. Two of the most important skills for students to learn during training are (a) to present a client effectively and (b) to record observations in an organized and efficient manner.

Guidelines for case presentation are in Figure 7.3. Greenberg and Jewett (1987) suggested the following guidelines for case presentation: (a) the case abstract including references should be no longer than 3½ typed pages, which may be single spaced; (b) the case history should include all relevant data; (c) the abstract should incorporate literature specific to the focus of the client; (d) a list of 3 to 10 pertinent recent references regarding the client in addition to a review article is recommended; (e) tables and graphs are helpful but not included in the 3½-page limit; and (f) audiovisual aids are helpful.

P. Schwartz, Fiddes, and Dempster (1987) described the *Case-Based Learning Day* (CBLD), which is a brief, self-contained exercise that is designed to introduce problem-based learning into a traditional curriculum. Clinical cases that raise important issues in the basic sciences are presented before

the students have had teaching on those topics in their regular courses. Students devise their own study plan while making use of printed and audiovisual resources of their choice and, if desired, faculty resource people. Their task is to apply basic science to help explain the underlying mechanisms of some aspects of the client's problems.

P. McLeod (1988) believes assessment of case reports permits evaluation of the student's information collection ability, clinical reasoning, and communication skills. Assessment of case reports may be useful educationally, and ratings should be obtained from several examiners on repeated occasions. See Figure 7.4 for a case reports assessment form, which ranks items from *poor* to *excellent*. A similar strategy would be to rank these items as *adequate* or *inadequate*.

Health science centers usually have meetings called grand rounds. Each session is devoted to specific clinical problems, cases, or approaches to diagnosis and treatment of certain disorders or certain case studies. Professionals from related disciplines or from the same discipline gather and exchange opinions on what was done, what might have been done, or what novel approach has been used, either to diagnose or to treat a given client. This concept has merit because it serves as a refresher, provides a forum for continuing education, and brings

---

Staffing Report

Client's Name: _____

Birthdate: _____

File: _____

Date of Staffing: _____

Date Report Received: _____

Reasons for Staffing: _____

_____

_____

Results of Staffing: _____

_____

_____

Approved by: _____
           Supervising Clinician

_____
           Clinician

Figure 7.2. Staffing report.

Do's and Don'ts of Staffing

Do

☐ Be sure that everyone knows all other team members and their professional affiliations.

☐ Provide basic information about the client in written form.

☐ Organize the discussion by providing a list of problems to be solved or areas to be considered. Set priorities. Discuss the most important issues first.

☐ Be sure everyone participates. Some individuals need to be encouraged to participate.

☐ Stimulate response and exchange. Nonverbal cues, such as nodding, frowning, or head shaking, are often clues that an individual needs to be called upon.

☐ Make certain everyone involved in a staffing both listens and talks.

☐ Summarize the discussion and state the decisions made, either at each juncture when the topic is to be changed, or at the end of staffing.

Don't

☐ Let members of the team just read their reports.

☐ Go around the table haphazardly asking individuals to say what they think. There is always a logical way to present information.

☐ Allow a staffing to get bogged down on minor or irrelevant issues.

Figure 7.3. Do's and don'ts of staffing. *Note.* Adapted from "Interdisciplinary Child Development Team: Team Issues and Training in Interdisciplinariness," by V. Holm and R. McMartin, 1978. In K. Allen, V. Holm, and R. Schiefelbusch (Eds.), *Early Intervention: A Team Approach* (pp. 97–102), Baltimore: University Park Press.

clinicians together at all levels to interact in a manner that promotes the betterment of everyone involved (Nodar, 1988).

mally. More formal oral reports include staffings and case presentations or grand rounds.

Summary

An oral report is any spoken factual statement that requires preparation and organization. Compared to its written equivalent, an oral report elicits direct listener response, is more personalized, may have a greater effect, and saves time. In contrast, a written report is easier to refine and organize, can be more complex, and can be reviewed easily. Depending on the situation, clinicians may give oral reports informally or for-

 ## Discussion Questions

1. How can speech–language pathologists and audiologists develop competence in listening?

2. What is the difference between informal and formal oral reports?

3. What are grand rounds?

4. Discuss the advantages and disadvantages of staffing.

Case Report Assessment

Student: _____   Clinician: _____

Reviewer: _____

	Poor	Fair	Average	Good	Excellent
I. Data Collection					
A. Abstract					
1. Accuracy of details	1	2	3	4	5
2. Clarity of characterization of symptoms	1	2	3	4	5
3. Completeness of information without omissions	1	2	3	4	5
4. Succinctness of descriptions	1	2	3	4	5
5. Chronologic description of sequence of events	1	2	3	4	5
B. History					
1. Accuracy of details	1	2	3	4	5
2. Completeness of information without omissions	1	2	3	4	5
3. Clarity of characterization of symptoms	1	2	3	4	5
4. Emphasis on relevant systems	1	2	3	4	5
II. Data Interpretation					
A. Identification of significant problems	1	2	3	4	5
B. Understanding of priorities in problem identification	1	2	3	4	5
C. Focus of discussion related to client	1	2	3	4	5
D. Succinctness of expression	1	2	3	4	5
III. Treatment					
A. Proper sequence of treatment	1	2	3	4	5
B. Appropriate treatment including family education	1	2	3	4	5
IV. Communication Skills					
A. Appropriate format and placement of information	1	2	3	4	5
B. Appropriate use of language and grammar	1	2	3	4	5
C. Ease of readability	1	2	3	4	5

Comments: _____

_____

_____

Grade: _____

Figure 7.4. Case report assessment.

Samples of Speech–Language–Hearing Reports

The diagnostic reports included in this appendix illustrate ways to apply the principles discussed in this book. The first example reports the assessment of a preschool child with delayed language acquisition. The second is a school-aged child with language deficits. The third describes assessment of a preschool child with a phonological disorder. In the fourth report, one of several approaches to reporting fluency assessment is described. The fifth example is an evaluation of a woman who has had laryngeal surgery for a condition caused by years of vocal abuse and misuse. The sixth is a report describing test results for a child with a submucous cleft palate and vocal nodules. The seventh example is the assessment of a 20-month-old child with a suspected hearing loss; it shows how to consider the need for auditory brainstem audiometry. The eighth report is about a teacher with a mixed motor speech disorder (apraxia and dysarthria); it illustrates how to address specific needs for further evaluation as well as general strategies for speech management. The ninth report concerns a young man with head injury and limited functional communication following an automobile accident. The tenth and eleventh reports are written in an abbreviated format similar to common practice in acute care and rehabilitation hospital settings and nursing homes. The tenth report is about a 69-year-old man who suffered a cerebralvascular accident (CVA) resulting in receptive and expressive aphasia. The eleventh report is about an 86-year-old woman with swallowing problems identified by the nursing staff while she was hospitalized with pneumonia. In all of the reports, names, dates, and specifics have been changed to protect client confidentiality.

The interested reader may find examples of reports elsewhere in the literature (Dalston, 1983; Dworkin & Hartman, 1988; Helm-Estabrooks & Aten, 1989; Lund & Duchan, 1988; Meitus, 1983; R. Miller & Groher, 1990).

Report 1: Delayed Speech and Language Acquisition—Preschool

Robert, a 2-year, 10-month-old male, was seen at the Speech, Language, and Hearing Center for a speech and language evaluation on July 1, 2001. He was referred by his pediatrician, George Smith, M.D. The mother is concerned about the child's "slow speech development." Following is a summary of the findings and recommendations based on the history, assessment results, and observations obtained during the evaluation.

History

Prenatal and birth histories as reported by Robert's mother were unremarkable. Medical history included fevers of 105 degrees secondary to chronic otitis media and bilateral myringotomies with ventilation tubes at 6 months. The mother reported that the tubes discharged 9 months later. Developmental milestones occurred within normal limits with the exception of speech and language acquisition, which was delayed. Robert said his first word at about 16 months and currently has a spoken vocabulary of approximately 30 to 40 words. He has recently begun using two-word combinations.

The child, along with two other toddlers, is cared for by his mother. His mother enjoys planning special play activities for the children each day.

Examination

Using visually reinforced responses, hearing screening was conducted with speech and pure tone stimuli in the sound field situation. Results show hearing sensitivity is within general normal limits for at least one ear. Immittance testing reveals normal traces and acoustic reflexes indicate normal middle ear function bilaterally.

The *Early Intervention Developmental Profile* (EIDP) was administered to obtain cognitive and linguistic developmental levels. On the cognition profile, Robert scored in the 24- to 27-month range, and on the language profile, he scored in the 20- to 23-month range. On the *Sequenced Inventory of Communication Development–Revised* (SICD–R), Robert achieved a receptive communication age of 24 months and an expressive communication age of 20 months. Scores on both measures are appreciably below expected performance, or greater than 1.5 standard deviations below the mean for his age. Language sampling analysis suggests an adequate range of pragmatic intentions (commenting, requesting, protesting, answering, labeling), a reduced range of semantic content categories, and a mean length of utterance of 1.12 morphemes. Robert's play skills and language use were assessed using Westby's *Symbolic Play Scale*. During spontaneous play, Robert asked for toys using single words, combined related toys (e.g., spoon and plate), and performed two sequential actions (e.g., putting block in truck, pushing truck), placing his development in symbolic play at approximately 22 to 24 months.

Throughout testing, Robert complied with familiar directions presented by the clinician or his mother but did not follow a new instruction. He had difficulty sustaining attention on any task and tended to move quickly from one activity to another.

Robert's speech is about 75% unintelligible. Based on spontaneous utterances, he has a reduced phonetic repertoire. Syllable structure is limited to CV (consonant–vowel) and CVCV (consonant–vowel–consonant–vowel) combinations.

During an oral mechanism screening, Robert had difficulty performing purposeful tongue movements. He protruded and depressed his tongue on command, but did not voluntarily lateralize it to either side. Although he could elevate the tongue sufficiently to produce the [t] and [d] phonemes in isolation, rapid tongue tip to alveolar ridge movements were slow.

Impressions

Robert presents a moderate to severe language delay and phonological disorder when his performance is compared to chronological age expectations. Contributing factors may include poor attending skills, limitations in motor control of the tongue, and the likelihood of fluctuating hearing levels associated with otitis media. Hearing at the time of the evaluation was normal in at least one ear as measured in the sound field situation. Tympanometry revealed normal middle ear status. Prognosis is deferred until Robert has had the benefit of several months of treatment.

Recommendations

Robert should be referred to a school-based preschool appraisal team to determine his eligibility for services. Treatment (or intervention) should emphasize language forms, functions, and meanings as well as facilitation of cognitive and social development and phonological awareness through pretend play activities simulating naturalistic contexts. After observing the activities in the clinical setting, Robert's mother should be assisted in implementing similar activities with Robert and the other toddlers she cares for in the home. Cognitive assessment should be completed as part of his preschool evaluation. Hearing should be monitored and reevaluated in 1 year or earlier at the parents' request.

Name, CCC-SLP; State Lic #, SLP
Program Director
Speech–Language Pathology

Name, CCC-A; State Lic #, A
Director of Audiology

Report 2: Language Deficit—School Age

Speech–Language Evaluation

Referral Information

John, an 11-year, 3-month-old male was seen for a speech and language evaluation at the Speech, Language, and Hearing Center on February 17. He was referred by Disability Determinations to assess his current speech and language skills. All information in this report was obtained from the case history, previous evaluations, parent interview, and results of the test battery.

History

Prenatal and birth history indicated that John was delivered by emergency C-section due to the cord being wrapped around his neck. His mother reported that John was not breathing at the time of birth, but was "quickly revived." John has had six sets of ventilation tubes for chronic middle ear infections and has respiratory problems that are controlled by medications. John is also on medication to control attention-deficit/hyperactivity disorder symptoms. Developmental milestones were all late, including speech development. According to the school system's pupil appraisal services, John was initially identified as an exceptional student in June 1992. He has received special education services since the completion of the initial evaluation, with several changes in exceptionality. He reportedly received speech therapy services in first and second grades, but was dismissed after meeting articulation goals. Language skills were never formally assessed. In 1998, John was reevaluated by the school system and identified as a student with a primary exceptionality of "emotional/behavioral disorders" and a secondary exceptionality of "learning disabilities." John is currently enrolled in the fourth grade and is having difficulty with all academic subjects except math. According to the school's standardized assessments, he has a significant deficit in writing skills, but is receiving no accommodations or modifications in his classroom. Peer relationships are reported to be poor and John is described by his mother as a "loner" who prefers to play on the computer at home.

Assessment Method

The following test battery was administered:

Pure Tone Audiometric Screening Re: ANSI Standards (1969)

Test of Auditory–Perceptual Skills–Revised (TAPS–R)

Peabody Picture Vocabulary Test–Third Edition (PPVT–III)

The Word–R Test

Clinical Evaluation of Language Fundamentals–Revised (CELF–R)

Informal Speech/Language Sample

Oral–peripheral Screening

Evaluation Results

John was accompanied to the evaluation by his mother. He entered the assessment willingly and was cooperative with all testing procedures. He occasionally asked the examiner for clarification when he did not understand a task, but seemed reluctant to say "I don't know" or guess when he did not know an answer. John was attentive throughout the evaluation, with no problems noted with impulsivity. He appeared to exercise his best effort and these results are believed to be an accurate assessment of his current speech and language skills.

A pure tone audiometric screening was completed under earphones using conventional response techniques. John passed all frequencies screened bilaterally at 20 dB.

The TAPS–R was administered to measure six areas of auditory perception. All subtest scaled scores were totaled and converted to an Auditory Perceptual Quotient of 104 (mean = 100) and an overall percentile rank of 59. Although this total score represents a performance in the average range, there was some discrepancy among individual subtest scores. John's performance on the word discrimination and most of the auditory memory tasks was at or above the mean for his age; however, his Auditory Processing subtest score was one standard deviation (*SD*) below the mean. This subtest requires the student to respond to thinking and reasoning questions.

The PPVT–III measures single-word receptive vocabulary. John obtained an age-equivalent score of 13 years, 2 months; a percentile rank of 73; and a standard score of 109 (mean = 100; *SD* = 15). This score was above the mean for current age expectations.

The Word–R tests expressive vocabulary and semantics. John's Total Test score of 67 was more than two standard deviations below the mean for his chronological age. He had the most difficulty with tasks that required a descriptive response or explanation.

Due to time constraints, only two subtests from the CELF–R were administered. These subtests were used to evaluate semantics, syntax, and morphology. John's performance on the Formulated Sentences subtest was one standard deviation below the mean for his age. Most of his errors were related to semantics (formulating a sentence with a clear and appropriate meaning) rather than word order or grammar.

During a conversation sample, John responded adequately to specific questions (requiring only a one- or two-word answer), but had difficulty participating expressively in dialogue. He did not initiate any spontaneous questions or comments and when asked open-ended questions, he gave only minimal responses, with no elaboration. Although a formal discourse analysis was not completed, John made numerous discourse errors across the domains of quantity, relation, and manner. He was also unable to organize a complete, coherent narrative (telling about a favorite movie) and made many ambiguous references, indicating problems with presuppositional meaning. Overall affect was flat, with minimal eye contact during conversation. John also blinked repeatedly and appeared to have other facial tics, which occurred when he was not speaking. When asked to write a sentence, he demonstrated significant difficulty with handwriting. There were no problems noted with syntax or grammar, but it was difficult to determine typical sentence length or complexity due to the limited conversational sample.

John's connected speech was characterized by some distortion of sibilants, accompanied by excess saliva. Intelligibility was good during structured tasks, but decreased in ongoing, connected speech. John sometimes repeated a phrase using a slower rate, which significantly improved his articulation. Oral structures were unremarkable; however, diadochokinetic rate was slow. Although some mild dysfluencies were noted, these appeared to be related to language difficulties rather than a primary fluency disorder. There was no accompanying tension or struggle with the dysfluencies and John seemed unaware of them. Voice quality was within normal limits.

Findings

Although John scored within the normal range on some standardized tests, he appears to have a moderate semantic–pragmatic language disorder when his overall performance is compared to current age expectations. John struggles with expressive semantics even though he has a good receptive vocabulary. He also appears to have weak auditory reasoning skills and poor pragmatics, most noticeable in his lack of conversational discourse skills. These weaknesses may account, at least in part, for John's difficulties with behavior and social skills and likely impact other academic areas as well. In addition, John's speech is characterized by a mild dysarthria which sometimes interferes with speech intelligibility. Birth history, developmental delays, questionable motor skills, speech characteristics, and possible facial tics all raise the question of neurological status.

Recommendations

1. It is recommended that John be referred to his primary care physician for consideration of a neurological evaluation.

2. It is recommended that John be referred for an occupational therapy evaluation to assess visual–perceptual and motor skills and to determine John's candidacy for using

assistive technology to complete written school assignments.

3. John should be reevaluated by his school system to determine his eligibility for occupational and speech therapy services. If he does not meet eligibility criteria, his parents may wish to pursue a trial period of therapy through a private agency.

4. Treatment goals should be directed toward improving semantic and pragmatic skills. Language therapy that uses a whole language approach, integrating reading, writing, and oral language, is recommended, using John's school curriculum in meaningful activities.

5. Additional testing in areas such as discourse analysis and situational problem solving may be helpful in further delineating pragmatic weaknesses. Pragmatic skills may be improved by working on problem-solving skills (e.g., "What would you do if . . . ?") and role-playing to practice appropriate social interactions and dialogue.

Name, CCC-SLP; State Lic #, SLP
Clinical Director
Speech–Language Pathology

Report 3: Phonological Disorder

David, a 4-year, 5-month-old male, was seen for a speech and language evaluation at the Speech, Language, and Hearing Center on May 16, 2001. He was referred by his preschool teacher, Jane Martin, to "determine the severity of his speech problem." His parents' primary concern is that David's speech may adversely affect his readiness for first grade. The following is a summary of findings and recommendations based on history, observation, and assessment information obtained during the evaluation.

History

Prenatal, birth, medical, and developmental histories provided by the mother were unremarkable. She reported that David has difficulty producing certain speech sounds such as "f" and "r," and that listeners unaccustomed to his speech have difficulty understanding him. David was further described as being active and alert. He attends a kindergarten for 4-year-olds in the morning and Kiddie Day Care in the afternoon.

Examination

David entered the testing situation willingly and cooperated enthusiastically in completing all tasks presented. His responses to pure tone stimuli presented at screening levels under earphones indicated hearing within normal limits bilaterally. Normal middle ear pressure and function were present on screening tympanometry.

David's scores on the subtests of the *Test of Language Development–Primary: Third Edition* that assess understanding and meaningful use of spoken words, grammar, and word discrimination (ability to distinguish between similar words) were all within normal limits for his age. During spontaneous speech, David used five- and six-word utterances mingled occasionally with complex sentences containing as many as 10 words. Semantics, syntax, and pragmatic skills were appropriate for his chronological age.

David's phonological error patterns were assessed using the *Assessment of Phonological Processes*. Among the many sound substitutions and occasional omissions were the following error patterns: reduction of consonant blends (e.g., "back" for *black*), stopping of fricatives in word-initial position (e.g., "pish" for *fish*), deaffrication of affricates in word-final position (e.g., "wat" for *watch*), and replacement of liquids with glides (e.g., "wing" for *ring*). Whole-word transcription revealed that he uses a broad phonetic inventory of speech sounds including stop sounds (/p/, /b/, /k/, /g/), fricative sounds (/s/, and /sh/), and nasal sounds (/m/, /n/, /ng/). In addition, he was stimulable with auditory and visual cues in producing consonant blends, fricatives, and affricates.

Analysis of articulation in connected speech revealed errors similar to those in single words. His speech intelligibility was judged to be 50%, but with careful listening in a known context, about 75% of the words spoken were intelligible. There is no evidence of oral structural or motor deficits. Speech fluency and vocal quality are judged normal.

Impressions

David has a moderate phonological disorder; etiology is unknown at this time. Based on his stimulability in correctly producing errored patterns and his cooperative behavior, prognosis for improvement appears good. Hearing as well as middle ear status are within normal limits on screening tests.

Recommendation

It is recommended that David be enrolled in a biweekly individual speech treatment program using a multiple phoneme phonologic production approach. His parents should be included in the treatment program so that transfer activities can be implemented from the onset.

Name, CCC-SLP; State Lic #, SLP
Clinical Supervisor

Report 4: Fluency Disorder

Julie, a 24-year-old female, was seen at the Speech, Language, and Hearing Center for a speech evaluation on November 14, 2001. She was referred by Myrtle Gifford, a vocational rehabilitation counselor. Julie's primary concern was that she "wants to join the Army and they won't accept a recruit with a speech problem." Following is a summary of the findings and recommendations based on the history, observations, and assessment results obtained during the evaluation.

History

Julie reports that she has stuttered since she was 4 years old and she recalls no unusual factors associated with the onset of her stuttering. She has never had speech treatment. The parochial school she attended did not provide speech services and financial limitations prevented her family from arranging for private treatment.

Julie described her health as "good." She is not taking medication. Other than an occasional cold, she has not had illnesses or accidents. According to Julie, her stuttering is similar in all speaking situations, except when she is relaxed she is more fluent. She further reports that her friends respond to her stuttering by being supportive and patient. However, she feels that her stuttering sometimes limits her social interaction with new acquaintances. Having completed an Associate Degree in dental hygiene, Julie works as a dental hygienist in a local dentist's office. She reports her stuttering occasionally interferes with her professional activity, particularly with male patients.

Examination

Julie responded to pure tone screening at 20 dBHL under earphones. Immittance testing revealed normal middle ear pressure and function bilaterally. Acoustic reflexes were present at screening levels. A screening of the oral mechanism reveals no structural or functional abnormalities. Based on informal screening, her articulation, voice quality, and language skills appear to be within normal limits.

The *Cooper Personalized Fluency Control Therapy–Assessment Protocol* was administered to assess fluency. The percentage of stuttered syllables averaged 10% across dialogue, monologue, and reading. An appreciable increase in stuttering frequency occurred under two conditions: (1) speaking in front of an audience of three unfamiliar adults, and (2) conversing during periods of communicative stress (time pressure, interruptions, and frequent clarification requests by the clinician). Types of dysfluencies included sound prolongations, part-word repetitions, and hard glottal productions of word-initial vowels. These moments of stuttering were accompanied by such accessory features as head jerks, poor eye contact, prolonged eyelid closures, and nostril flaring. The duration of stuttering instances ranged from 2 to 13 seconds with an average of 4 seconds. Consequently, Julie's speech rate was 120 syllables per minute. Periods of fluency, however, were characterized by a rapid speech rate (230 syllables per minute) and an "unnatural" quality of monotonic intonation.

Using scaled responses and anecdotal ratings, Julie identified 21 of 50 situations as ones she would avoid or prefer to avoid. There were several indications of a negative attitude about the effects of her stuttering. On a scale of 1 to 5 with 5 being *most severe,* Julie rated the severity of her stuttering as 2.5, whereas the clinician's severity rating of her stuttering was 3.5.

Julie's response to trial treatment was good. When using easy onset of phonation in the production of words, her percentage of stuttering was reduced to 1%. She easily replicated a model of prolonged speech rate (one syllable per second), and accessory features were eliminated when speaking in this manner.

Impressions

Julie has a moderate to severe fluency disorder that appears to be socially and vocationally disabling. Julie appears shy and withdrawn, yet her apparent motivation to improve speech, along with her ability to modify fluency using easy onset of phonation, suggests a favorable prognosis for improvement. Hearing and middle ear status were within normal limits on screening measures.

Recommendations

Julie should enroll in both individual and group treatment. Individual treatment should focus on the use of specific fluency-enhancing speech strategies and accompanying transfer activities. She also should consider attending a stuttering support group to facilitate self-confidence and establish a network among others who stutter.

Name, CCC-SLP; State Lic #, SLP
Speech–Language Pathologist

Report 5: Phonatory Voice Disorder

Ms. Josephine Jones, a 60-year-old female, was seen for a voice evaluation at the Speech, Language, and Hearing Center on February 14, 2001. She was referred by Dr. Donald Martin, M.D., otolaryngologist, for treatment following laryngeal surgery. Following is a summary of the findings and recommendations based on history and assessment results collected in this evaluation.

History

According to Ms. Jones, a homemaker who lives alone, Dr. Martin diagnosed vocal fold lesions or leukoplakia. He stripped her left vocal fold on January 6, 2001, and reported that the right vocal fold was reddened and edematous. She was placed on complete vocal rest for 2 weeks during which time she communicated using a pad and pencil. After 2 weeks she resumed talking for limited periods of time while being careful not to abuse her voice. She no longer limits her speech and reports less awareness of vocal abuses.

Ms. Jones reported a history of voice problems throughout much of her life. Her voice has always been low pitched for her age and gender but has become even lower during the past few years. Fifteen years ago, she consulted an otolaryngologist about chronic phonatory hoarseness. Medication was prescribed and her voice improved somewhat. Ms. Jones did not return for the recommended follow-up.

For many years, Ms. Jones smoked two or three packs of cigarettes daily. She quit smoking after her recent surgery, but reports that she now experiences increased nervousness. She says she "talks a lot, but never in noisy conditions or for long periods of time." Ms. Jones prefers to spend her leisure time reading or talking in small groups while playing bridge. She reports that her throat has been sore since the surgery, particularly since she resumed talking after the prescribed vocal rest.

Examination

Ms. Jones failed a pure tone hearing screening bilaterally at 20 dBHL at several frequencies in each ear. Immittance screening revealed normal traces and acoustic reflexes for both ears.

Assessment of the voice parameters revealed marked dysphonia with occasional pitch judged low considering her age and gender. Despite adequate respiratory driving pressure (7.5 cm H_2O of pressure for 10 seconds), Ms. Jones was unable to sustain phonation of "ah" for more than 3 seconds. The VisiPitch was used to assess acoustic correlates of pitch and quality. In connected speech, fundamental frequency was from 101 Hz to 188 Hz, with an average frequency or habitual pitch of 136 Hz. This measure is approximately 1.5 standard deviations below the mean for adult females her age. A reduced phonational frequency of 95 Hz to 320 Hz was obtained by having Ms. Jones produce the highest and lowest sounds she could using a singing scale in a stepwise fashion. The abnormally high frequency perturbation rating of 2.6 was consistent with the perception of phonatory roughness. Regarding intensity, amplitude averaged 30 dB, with a rapid decrease during vowel phonation and connected speech. With cuing, maximum intensity was 65 dB.

Using facilitating approaches such as easy onset phonation and chewing combined with the VisiPitch for visual feedback, Ms. Jones increased the duration of phonation to 9 seconds and inconsistently produced sustained phonation with a perturbation rating of 1.2 and an average frequency of 170 Hz. When encouraged to speak with greater lung volume, vocal intensity averaged 37 dB. These measures suggest voice quality, intensity, and habitual pitch that are essentially normal for a female her chronological age.

Articulation, language, and fluency skills were normal.

Impressions

Ms. Jones has a phonatory dysphonia that makes her voice so weak in intensity that she has difficulty communicating in other than quiet, small groups. Because she has quit smoking and can increase the duration and intensity of phonation while improving pitch and quality using the VisiPitch, Ms. Jones appears to be a good candidate for short-term voice treatment. Hearing screening suggests a possible hearing problem. Middle ear status was normal on screening tympanometry.

Recommendations

Ms. Jones should be enrolled in voice treatment emphasizing awareness and implementation of good vocal habits, increasing the duration and integrity of phonation, while improving quality and pitch using visual feedback. She should be scheduled for a complete audiological evaluation. Continued otolaryngological follow-up is recommended.

_____

Name, CCC-SLP; State Lic #, SLP
Speech–Language Pathologist

Report 6: Resonance Voice Disorder

Homer, a 4-year, 9-month-old boy, was seen for speech and language evaluation at the Speech, Language, and Hearing Center on January 15, 2001. Homer's mother reported that, "He is receiving speech therapy and has a bifid uvula." She further described nasal emission and hypernasal speech as well as numerous articulation errors when describing Homer's speech.

In addition, she stated that since Homer has been attending speech therapy, the nasal emission has diminished but continues to occur in rapid connected speech. The purpose of this examination is to determine the need for further assessment of velopharyngeal function.

History

Homer has medically diagnosed vocal nodules. Complete birth, medical, and developmental histories are reported in previous evaluation reports.

Examination

On the *Receptive One-Word Picture Vocabulary Test,* Homer achieved a standard score of 96, which translates to the age equivalent of 4 years, 7 months. The *Structured Photographic Expressive Language Test–II* (SPELT–II) is a standardized measure for production of specific morphological and syntactical structures; Homer's score was 5. The mean score for a child of his chronological age is 22.39. On the *Oral Language Imitation Sentence Test–Stage III,* Homer's mean length of imitative utterance was 5.2. He was able to accurately imitate most linguistic structures, although sentence length was sometimes reduced. Analysis of a spontaneous language sample corroborated findings from the SPELT–II. Based on an analysis of a spontaneous language sample, Homer's mean length of utterance was 3.25. He used present progressive verbs (e.g., *smiling*) and prepositions (e.g., *in, on, under*), but did not use past tense verbs in the sample.

The *Templin-Darley Tests of Articulation* (TDTA) is a series of single-word tests of articulation. The *Iowa Pressure Articulation Test* (IPAT), a 43-item subtest of the TDTA, assesses the adequacy of oral pressure for speech sound production and, thus, inferentially the adequacy of velopharyngeal closure during speech. During the production of pressure consonants on the IPAT, nasal emissions, weak pressure consonants, and substitution of glottal stops were the primary error types. On McWilliams and Philips's *Weighted Values for Speech Symptoms Associated with VPI,* which is based on symptoms heard or seen during speech, Homer's cumulative score was 12. A score of 7 or above suggests velopharyngeal incompetency.

Homer's spontaneous speech was characterized by nasal emission, hypernasality, nasal grimacing, hoarseness, breathiness, and glottal stop substitutions. The Nasometer was used to further identify the presence of excessive nasality. When the mean scores for nonnasal and nasal reading passages were compared, there was no significant difference (9.41) between the mean scores, suggesting the presence of hypernasality during speech.

Examination of oral structure revealed a bifid uvula, hypertrophied palatine tonsils, and a bony deficiency on the posterior margin of the hard palate.

Homer passed hearing screening bilaterally. Otoscopy revealed the presence of ventilation tubes. The PE tube in the right ear was coming out; therefore, immittance testing was not performed on the right ear. Immittance screening indicated a nonpatent ventilation tube in the left ear. Normal middle ear pressure and function were found in that ear.

Impressions

Homer has a delay in expressive language development including a moderately severe articulation problem. His voice is characterized by the presence of moderate hoarseness and mild to moderate hypernasality. It is possible that the dysphonia has developed as a nonadaptive compensation for velopharyngeal insufficiency. Hearing was in normal limits on a screening test. Visual examination and tympanometry indicated ventilation tubes are present but may not be functional.

Recommendations

Based on the findings of the evaluation, the following are recommended:

1. Behavioral speech treatment pending consideration of medical management of the velopharynx.
2. Radiographic or endoscopic evaluation, or both, of velopharyngeal closure would be diagnostically beneficial.
3. Laryngoscopic reevaluation is warranted in view of the moderate phonatory hoarseness.
4. Continued speech and language treatment to improve his use of morphological and syntactical structures and articulation skills.
5. Evaluation of the status of ventilation tubes by Homer's otolaryngologist.

Name, CCC-SLP; State Lic #, SLP
Speech–Language Pathologist

Name, CCC-A; State Lic #, A
Audiologist

Report 7: Hearing Impairment

Karen, age 20 months, received hearing evaluations at the Speech, Language, and Hearing Center on October 4, 11, and November 8, 2001. She was referred by the Regional Deaf Center to determine her hearing sensitivity.

History

Prenatal and birth histories provided by the mother were unremarkable. Motor milestones have been met within normal limits; however, Karen has no spoken words at this time. She appears to hear some sounds, but does not demonstrate consistent comprehension of speech. She has a history of frequent ear infections prior to the insertion of ventilating tubes on June 10, 2001. She is scheduled to see her otolaryngologist for regular followup visits every 3 to 4 months. Since the insertion of tubes, she is demonstrating more responsiveness to sound but still has no spoken words.

Examination

Hearing testing was done in a sound field setting using visual reinforcement techniques to obtain responses to warbled pure tone and speech stimuli. On October 4, 2001, Karen responded inconsistently to warbled pure tone stimuli. A speech awareness threshold was obtained at 55 dBHL. Immittance measurements revealed a normal trace for the left ear and a functioning ventilation tube or perforated eardrum in the right ear. A ventilation tube was visualized in the right tympanic membrane on otoscopic inspection. The left eardrum appeared to be intact. Since the test results were inconclusive, she was scheduled for further testing.

On October 11, 2001, hearing testing was again completed in a sound field setting. A speech awareness threshold of 25 dBHL was obtained; however, responses to warbled pure tone stimuli were inconsistent between 45 and 50 dBHL for air conduction. Bone conduction testing could not be completed because she would not tolerate the bone conduction oscillator. Immittance measurements and otoscopic examination were unchanged. Findings on the right were consistent with a functioning ventilation tube. There was no evidence of active middle ear difficulty on the right side.

The last evaluation was completed on November 8, 2001. Responses to warbled pure tone stimuli were consistent at 45 to 50 dBHL for air conduction. However, Karen responded several times to pure tones presented at 20 to 25 dBHL. Speech awareness was established at 25 dBHL. Immittance measurements and otoscopic examination results remained unchanged.

Karen imitated the examiner during play activity (e.g., throwing a ball to knock down bowling pins) and used gestures and vocalizations effectively to ask for specific toys that were out of her reach. It was difficult to establish even brief eye contact with her; she was very distracted by her surroundings in the clinical setting. She would not imitate the examiner's repetitive syllables or monosyllabic words for toys she was playing with (e.g., "ba, ba, ba" or "ball").

Impressions

The possibility of a mild to moderate hearing loss could not be ruled out on the basis of this series of audiometrics. The immittance measurements and otoscopic inspection suggested that Karen does not have a middle ear problem in the left ear at this time. She does appear to have a functioning ventilation tube in the right eardrum.

Recommendations

1. Karen's hearing should be evaluated using brainstem audiometrics. This objective technique is used to establish hearing levels in individuals who do not or cannot respond consistently to auditory stimuli during testing.
2. She should return to her otolaryngologist for the recommended follow-up medical assessments.
3. A speech and language evaluation is recommended.

Name, CCC-A; State Lic #, A
Director of Audiology

Report 8: Motor Speech Disorder

Initially evaluated on February 5, 2001, 29-year-old Laura sought treatment for "nasal speech." A special education teacher with a master's degree from the state university, Laura is seeking help because her principal recently criticized her speech in her annual performance appraisal.

History

Laura related a long history of speech therapy in elementary school focusing on language, articulation, and fluency. She further related that her early development was characterized by poor overall coordination and difficulty learning to write, drooling, regurgitation of liquids, poor visual perception, difficulty learning to read, and poor articulation. She was dismissed as corrected from treatment prior to entering high school.

She has had no serious illness and reported that she is generally very healthy. She eats a regular diet but reported that she is a very slow and somewhat messy eater.

Examination

On the *Dworkin-Culatta Oral Mechanism Examination*, Laura had poor muscle control on the left side of the face and tongue. Lingual diadochokinesis (repetitive tongue movements) and sequential syllable rates were slow. In attempting to complete volitional tongue movements, Laura exhibited a lack of speed, range, strength, and precision of movement. Some drooling was observed, and labial diadochokinesis (repetitive lip movement) was slow and labored. Laura's palate was high and narrowly arched. She has a Class II (distoclusion or overbite) malocclusion and the upper right lateral incisor is missing. During eating and swallowing, food manipulation was adequate but with some output of crumbs to her lips and chin during mastication. She swallowed very small quantities of liquid at a time.

On the sentence portion of the *Templin-Darley Tests of Articulation*, no articulation errors were identified. However, her resonance was mildly hypernasal and nasal grimacing was evident during production of pressure consonants. During connected speech, she had glottal air stoppages resulting in disruption of speech flow. Prosody (the intonation and stress patterns or melody of speech) was characterized by equalized stress and reduced speech rate.

Laura's responses to items on the *Frenchay Dysarthria Assessment* revealed below normal function of the drool reflex and slow laryngeal timing and tongue elevation.

Pure tone audiological assessment revealed hearing within normal limits. Immittance testing revealed normal middle ear pressure and function. However, her word recognition in sound field was 48% at a +10 signal to noise ratio, which is significantly low and suggestive of possible central auditory involvement.

Impressions

Laura has a mild to moderate motor speech disorder of undetermined etiology. The test results indicate the presence of a flaccid dysarthria characterized by hypernasality, glottal air stoppages, and prosodic breakdown, primarily involving speech rhythm and rate. Peripheral hearing acuity was normal, but testing in noise suggests a possible central problem. She may be experiencing some difficulty in swallowing thin liquids.

Recommendations

Laura should be scheduled for the following: (1) a complete neurological examination to determine the possibility of cranial nerve involvement; (2) a radiographic or endoscopic study of the velopharyngeal mechanism; (3) a complete swallow study; (4) speech treatment to increase strength and specificity of articulator movement, provide practice in patterning and pacing articulator movements during speech, and pending the outcome of a swallow study, may include strategies for swallowing safely; and (5) additional assessment of central auditory function which can be incorporated into her treatment program.

Name, CCC-SLP; State Lic #, SLP
Speech–Language Pathologist

Name, CCC-A; State Lic #, A
Audiologist

Report 9: Traumatic Brain Injury

Joseph, a 26-year-old male, was seen for a speech and language evaluation at the Speech, Language, and Hearing Center on April 21, 2001. He has deficits in communication, cognition, attention, and social judgment, resulting from a traumatic brain injury. Joseph has had previous evaluations and treatment in acute care and rehabilitation settings. The purpose of this evaluation is to determine Joseph's communicative status and if additional speech–language treatment is warranted.

History

Joseph was discharged from the army because of physical and communication deficits secondary to a left depressed skull fracture caused by an automobile accident in June 1997. He sustained left frontal cerebral lesions along with diffuse axonal injury of the white matter. He was in a coma for 24 hours and had posttraumatic amnesia.

Prior to the brain injury, Joseph indicated that his communication, thinking, and socialization were "normal." His health was generally good. He was a nonsmoker who did not partake of recreational drugs. Alcohol consumption was described as light. Following graduation from high school, Joseph completed 1½ years at Community College. His studies focused on electronics and business administration. He decided to enlist in the army to further his education while receiving financial support.

According to Joseph's parents, his immediate posttrauma signs included a right hemiplegia, disorientation, loss of mem-

ory, and impaired attention. He was aphonic and experienced some swallowing difficulty. Four months posttrauma, Joseph understood general conversation about familiar topics, could read for comprehension various familiar words and phrases related to objects or daily needs, and could select the correct answer to questions from several choices.

At that time, he used a communication notebook that included a calendar, his daily schedule, and words and phrases that conveyed his basic communication needs.

Upon discharge from the hospital in March 1998, Joseph had improved in visual, memory, and graphic skills but continued to have a motor speech disorder. An electronic augmentative communication system was tailored to his linguistic, motor, and cognitive skills and he received training in using the device. Joseph lived with his parents and sister until his admission to the Rehabilitation Center in July 2000.

Subsequent rehabilitation included speech, physical, and occupational therapies. He had slow but noticeable improvement in speech production and ambulation. His use of the augmentative communication device was recently discontinued because he now wants to rely on oral communication for his daily communication.

Examination

Joseph was cooperative during a lengthy testing session. He displayed excellent frustration tolerance and physical endurance. However, a lack of insight for some of the higher level thinking tasks and a degree of denial regarding his deficits were noted. For example, he provided simplistic answers to complex problem-solving tasks while conveying his conviction that the answers were accurate.

Attention

Joseph had some focusing difficulty when perceiving alternatives and reflecting on responses. Evaluation and planning skills were appropriate. Occasional distractibility resulting in disrupted concentration was noted. Responses were excessively tangential and revised on difficult subtests.

Memory

Joseph had moderate difficulty storing and retrieving information from immediate recall on the Immediate Memory subtest of the *Ross Information Processing Assessment–Second Edition* (RIPA–2). He had mild difficulty recalling and receiving information requiring organization on the RIPA–2 Organization Subtest, and moderate difficulty in perception, discrimination, sequencing, and recalling information on the RIPA–2 Auditory Processing and Retention Subtest. Informal observation of recent memory, remote memory, and recall of general information was appropriate. Episodic memory was not assessed.

Language

Rate of auditory processing was inconsistent, usually being adequate, sometimes slightly delayed, and occasionally markedly reduced. Joseph demonstrated low average skills in interpreting factual information presented in spoken paragraphs on the *Clinical Evaluation of Language Fundamentals–Revised* (CELF–R). He occasionally asked for repetitions to clarify. His score reflected very low skills (greater than two standard deviations below the mean) on the *Test of Linguistic Concepts: Understanding Ambiguous Sentences*. He had difficulty perceiving alternatives, although evaluation and planning skills remained intact. Severe difficulties with reading simple instructions, writing, solving simple math problems, and telling time were identified by his performance on the *Assessment of Language-Related Function Activities*.

Expressively, interpersonal pragmatic skills were impaired. Conversational responses were frequently tangential and Joseph had difficulty elaborating on a topic and shifting registers. Sometimes, for example, he produced inappropriately sarcastic remarks, suggesting difficulty in controlling suprasegmental (speech intonation, rhythm, and stress) cues. Syntax was generally well formed, but there were instances of paraphasias and "empty" content. Narratives were replete with referencing errors and lacked cohesion. Joseph had considerable difficulty producing figurative reference. For instance, when asked to generate two different meanings, he needed 21 minutes to generate two meanings for 10 sentences.

Speech Production

Joseph has a mild to moderate dysarthria. Articulation errors included deletion of unstressed syllables, omission of final consonants, and difficulty producing polysyllabic words. The *Assessment of Intelligibility of Dysarthric Speech* yielded an intelligibility rating of 70% for single words and 82% for sentences. Speech rate (116 syllables per minute) was reduced. Prosody was characterized by excess stress and prolonged intervals. Joseph's voice was moderately dysphonic, characterized by an abnormally low pitch, clavicular breathing, inappropriate phrasing, audible inspiration, glottal fry, reduced pitch range, and a strained, strangled quality. Conversational speech was about 75% intelligible with contextual cues.

Oral Peripheral Examination

Examination revealed normal structure but signs of unilateral motor weakness. There was a slight right side facial weakness when smiling and deviation of the tongue to the left upon protrusion. Joseph had difficulty making rapid discrete lingual movements. Diadochokinetic rates (repetitive sound and syllable productions) were slow and laborious. Velar elevation was symmetrical. A dysphagia screening suggested swallowing is within normal limits.

Hearing

Joseph failed a pure tone hearing screening for the frequencies 1000 and 2000 Hz at 20 dBHL bilaterally.

Impressions

Joseph presents moderate to severe deficits in language, articulation, voice, memory, and attention. Although he has made considerable improvement in the past 2 years, his difficulties continue to interfere with vocational and social interaction. Considering Joseph's motivation, the prognosis for some continued improvement is guardedly favorable. Hearing screening suggests a possible hearing problem.

Recommendations

Joseph should be enrolled in a speech and language treatment program focusing on articulation and voice, pragmatic aspects of communication, and figurative language use. Audiological evaluation should also be scheduled. Laryngeal structure and function should be assessed by an ear–nose–throat physician. Information from videonasoendoscopy and stroboscopy would provide helpful diagnostic information.

Name, CCC-SLP; State Lic #, SLP
Speech–Language Pathologist

Report 10: Adult Post-Stroke with Aphasia

Name: Hank Smith

Date of Evaluation: 9/21/2001

Date of Birth: 08/17/1932

Facility: Community General Hospital

Physician: Richard E. Martin, M.D.

☒ Inpatient   ☐ Outpatient

Primary Diagnosis (Onset Date): 9/16/2001; CVA Left Hemisphere

Communication Disorder (Onset Date): 9/16/2001; receptive and expressive aphasia

ICD–9# 784.3

Precautionary Information: Right hemiparesis

Physician Order: 9/20/2001; speech evaluation and treatment according to care plan

Payor Source: Medicare

Prior Function

Until the time of the CVA on 9/16/2001, Mr. Smith was the chief comptroller for the Galaxy Computer Resources Corporation. During his 5-day hospitalization, he has improved in alertness, orientation, and motor skills according to the family and nursing staff.

Initial Assessment

Based on a chart review, observations by nursing staff and family, interview with the patient, informal measures, and selected portions of the *Western Aphasia Battery*, results are as follows:

Verbal and Language Skills: Communicates wants and needs at a conversational level; speech is 90% intelligible; word finding difficulties on about 50% of words attempted; decreased ability in convergent naming and tangential communication; excessive attention to detail instead of the main idea of a conversation.

Pragmatics: Eye contact, topic maintenance, and turn taking were adequate.

Auditory Comprehension: Answered simple questions and followed multiple commands.

Cognition: Oriented when speaking to one person at a time; deficits in problem solving (about 60% accuracy); some difficulty with attention and concentration.

Reading: Comprehends only about 60% of passages from the newspaper.

Writing: Is right handed so experiencing difficulty writing due to right hemiparesis involving the right arm.

Hearing: In seminoisy environment, asked for repetition during conversation.

Oral Structure and Function: Oral musculature appeared normal in structure, function, and symmetry; he has his own teeth.

Swallowing: Observation of consumption of a regular diet including thin liquids revealed no overt swallowing difficulties.

Impressions and Recommendations

Mr. Smith is experiencing deficits in verbal language, reading comprehension, cognition, writing, and hearing. Speech and language treatment is indicated as a medical necessity to increase functional communication, comprehension, orientation, and safety in his home environment upon discharge. Prognosis appears good based on his level of motivation, his ability to attend to tasks for adequate periods of time, and family's dedication to support the program. Treatment should be scheduled daily for 4 weeks. In addition, a complete audiological evaluation is recommended.

Name, CCC-SLP; State Lic #, SLP
Speech–Language Pathologist

Report 11: Adult with Dysphagia

Name: Elvia Muñoz

Date of Evaluation: 2/7/2000

Date of Birth: 9/2/1913

Facility: General Care Center

Physician: Elvis A. Rock, M.D.

☒ Inpatient   ☐ Outpatient

Primary Diagnosis (Onset Date): 1/25/2000; Pneumonia

Communication Disorder (Onset Date): 1/25/2000; Dysphagia

ICD–9# 787.2

Precautionary Information: Left side neglect

Physician Order: 2/4/2000; speech evaluation and treatment according to care plan

Payor Source: Medicare

Prior Function

Ms. Muñoz, an 86-year-old resident of General Care Center, had a CVA on 10/19/1999. At that time left-sided weakness with no swallowing difficulties and adequate vocal quality and intensity were noted. While hospitalized (admitted 1/25/2000) with pneumonia, nursing staff reported patient was coughing on liquids. Ms. Muñoz wears bilateral in-the-ear hearing aids and is followed at the G. W. Katze Speech and Hearing Clinic.

Initial Assessment

Ms. Muñoz was observed eating a regular diet. She used chin tucks while drinking liquids. Her vocal quality prior to drinking liquids was hoarse and weak in intensity. After drinking liquids, her voice had a wet quality. After coughing, clearing the throat, and swallowing at request of clinician, the wet vocal quality decreased. She routinely washed down bites of solid food with liquids. Ms. Muñoz understood the clinician without difficulty while wearing her hearing aids.

Clinical Impressions

Changes in vocal quality and reports of coughing on liquids places Ms. Muñoz at risk for aspiration. Since she washed down each bite of solid food with liquids, she may have a decreased swallow reflex triggered only after liquid presentation. Prognosis for maximizing efficiency and safety of the swallow appears good.

Recommendations

1. Exercises to strengthen laryngeal and oral musculature.
2. Instruction to the patient, nursing staff, and the family on swallowing precautions to decrease risk of aspiration, including procedures for cuing Ms. Muñoz to utilize chin tucks and use double swallow and cough to clear the airway when needed during swallowing of liquids.
3. Continued management of hearing problems at the Katze Clinic.

Name, CCC-SLP; State Lic #, SLP
Speech–Language Pathologist

Samples of Problem-Oriented Reports

The Problem Oriented Reports (POR) included in this appendix illustrate ways to apply the principles discussed in this book. Some of the clients presented in Appendix A are used again in this appendix so the reader may compare the same information provided in a traditional reporting style and in the POR format.

 Sample 1

Client in Report 1, Appendix A

Robert, age 2 years, 10 months

Problem List

Delayed speech and language acquisition

Subjective

Chronic otitis media with ventilation tubes at 6 months. Normal motor development. Delayed speech development: first word 16 months; currently has 10-word spoken vocabulary; does not combine words.

Objective

Hearing: Responses to speech and pure tone stimuli via sound field suggest normal hearing in at least one ear. Immittance revealed normal traces and acoustic reflexes.

Language: EIDP: Cognition 24- to 27-month level and language 20- to 23-month level.

SICD: Receptive age 28 months and expressive communication age 24 months.

Symbolic Play Scale: Symbolic play development at 17- to 19-month level.

Language sample: MLU of 1.12 morphemes

Played meaningfully with toys but did not follow directions.

Briefly attended to tasks; he did not visually focus on materials or remain in proximity of the examiner.

Speech: Utterances 75% unintelligible; used jargon and gestures.

Oral peripheral screening: Difficulty with purposeful tongue movements.

Assessment

Moderate language delay and phonological disorder.

Plan

1. Enroll in a structured preschool speech–language treatment program.

2. Continue to observe to further assess level of speech–language performance.

3. Refer to school system for complete evaluation.

4. Explain to parents that (1) delayed speech and language may result from several factors and that cognitive assessment would be diagnostically beneficial, and (2) further speech–language assessment will aid in establishing diagnosis and prognosis.

5. Reevaluate his speech, language, and hearing in 1 year or earlier at the parents' request.

Name, CCC-SLP; State Lic #, SLP
Speech–Language Pathologist

Sample 2

Client in Report 5, Appendix A

Ms. Josephine Jones, age 60 years

Problem List

1. Dysphonia
2. Possible hearing loss

Problem 1—Dysphonia

Subjective

History of voice problems including low pitch. Formerly smoked 2 to 3 packs of cigarettes daily. Described self as nervous and talking a lot.

Objective

Left vocal fold stripped in January 2001; two weeks vocal rest. Has not returned for ENT follow-up. Analysis of voice revealed marked dysphonia with occasional low pitch. Failed hearing screening (see Problem 2).

Assessment

Phonatory dysphonia

Plan

1. Obtain ENT consult.

2. Explain to client that dysphonia may result from several factors, and that continued ENT follow-up is necessary.
3. Identification and elimination of vocal abuse(s).

Problem 2—Possible Hearing Loss

Subjective

Client does not seem aware of hearing difficulties.

Objective

Failed pure tone hearing screening.

Assessment

Possible hearing loss.

Plan

1. Explain to client that results suggest need for audiological evaluation.
2. Obtain audiological evaluation.

Name, CCC-SLP; State Lic #, SLP
Speech–Language Pathologist

Sample 3 (SOAP Format)

Client in Report 5, Appendix A

Ms. Josephine Jones, age 60 years

Date	Problem	Status Outset	Team Agenda	Intervention Plan
January 14–19, 2001	Dysphonia		ENT consult	
	Low Pitch	$F_0 = 136$ Hz	SLP	VisiPitch
	Roughness	Perturbation Rating = 2.6	SLP	Prolonged "ah" 3- or 4-word sentences Easy onset; respiratory control
	Vocal abuses	Talks excessively	SLP	Checklist for usual daily speaking activities
	Hearing loss	Failed screening	Audiologist	Audiological assessment

Sample 4

Client in Report 6, Appendix A

Homer, age 4 years, 9 months

Problem List

1. Misarticulation and hypernasality
2. Phonatory hoarseness
3. Possible delayed expressive language acquisition

Problem 1—Misarticulation and Hypernasality

Subjective

Mother reported that Homer is receiving speech therapy; has a bifid uvula; speech characterized by nasal emission, hypernasality, and numerous articulation errors. Nasal emission has diminished since began speech therapy but occurs in rapid connected speech.

Objective

Iowa Pressure Articulation Test: nasal emissions, weak pressure consonants, and substitution of glottal stops.

McWilliams and Philips's *Weighted Values for Speech Symptoms Associated with VPI* = Score of 12 (7 or above suggests velopharyngeal incompetency).

Speech sample: nasal emission, hypernasality, nasal grimacing, hoarseness, breathiness, and glottal stop substitutions.

Nasometer: no significant difference (9.41) between the mean scores for nonnasal and nasal reading passages, suggesting presence of hypernasality during speech.

Oral structure examination: bifid uvula, hypertrophied tonsils, and a bony deficiency on the posterior margin of the hard palate.

Hearing screening: hearing sensitivity normal bilaterally; ventilation tube in right ear appears to be coming out. PE tube in left ear is intact and normal middle ear pressure and function were found in that ear.

Assessment

Moderate to severe articulation problem; mild to moderate hypernasality.

Plan

1. Obtain direct examination of velopharyngeal function (i.e., radiographic and/or endoscopic evaluation).
2. Explain to parents that misarticulation and hypernasality may result from velopharyngeal incompetence and that direct examination is necessary.

Problem 2—Phonatory Hoarseness

Subjective

The parents do not appear aware of the hoarseness or vocal abuse(s). The mother reported that Homer has medically diagnosed vocal nodules.

Objective

Phonatory hoarseness is present on single words and in connected speech.

Assessment

Phonatory quality is moderately hoarse.

Plan

1. Obtain laryngoscopic reevaluation.
2. Discuss with parents that hoarseness may result from vocal nodules or velopharyngeal incompetence.
3. Suggest approaches for identifying vocal abuse(s).

Problem 3—Possible Delayed Expressive Language Acquisition

Subjective

The parents do not appear aware of language difficulties.

Objective

Receptive One-Word Picture Vocabulary Test standard score of 96, age equivalent of 4 years, 7 months; *Structured Photographic Expressive Language Test–II* (SPELT–II), a standardized measure of morphological and syntactical structures, score was 5 (mean score for a child his chronological age is 22.39); *Oral Language Imitation Sentence Test–Stage III:* mean length of imitative utterance was 5.2 (he accurately imitated most linguistic structures, but sentence length was sometimes reduced). Based on an analysis of a spontaneous speech sample, Homer's mean length of utterance was 3.25. He used present progressive verbs (e.g., *smiling*) and prepositions (e.g., *in, on, under*), but did not use past tense verbs in the sample.

Assessment

Delayed expressive language development, perhaps secondary to Problem #1.

Plan

1. Discuss current levels of language performance with parents.
2. Speech and language treatment to improve his use of morphological and syntactical structures and articulation skills.

Sample 5

Client in Report 7, Appendix A

Karen, age 20 months

Problem List

Possible hearing loss

Subjective

No spoken words; appears to hear some sounds; does not consistently comprehend speech. Chronic otitis media with ventilation tubes.

Objective

Responded inconsistently to warbled pure tones; Speech awareness threshold established at 25 dBHL. Imitated motor activities during play but would not imitate syllables or mono-syllabic words. Used gestures and vocalizations to ask for toys.

Assessment

Possible hearing loss

Plan

1. Obtain brainstem audiometrics.
2. Obtain ENT consult.
3. Obtain speech–language pathology consult.
4. Explain to parents that brainstem audiometry, and consults by ENT and speech–language pathology are necessary in establishing a plan of management.

_____
Name, CCC-A; State Lic #, A
Audiologist

Sample 6 (SOAP Format)

Client in Report 11, Appendix A

Ms. Elvia Muñoz, age 86 years

Subjective

CVA on 10/19/1999 with left-sided weakness but no reported swallowing difficulties; hospitalized 1/25/2000 with pneumonia; while hospitalized nursing staff observed coughing on liquids. Ms. Muñoz has a diagnosed hearing loss and wears bilateral in-the-ear hearing aids. She is followed audiometrically on a regular basis at the G. W. Katze Speech and Hearing Clinic.

Objective

Eats regular diet using chin tucks while drinking liquids; vocal quality prior to drinking liquids is hoarse and weak in intensity; wet vocal quality after drinking liquids; after coughing, throat clearing, and swallowing after drinking liquids, the wet vocal quality decreases; routinely washes down bites of solid food with liquids. Ms. Muñoz was wearing her hearing aids at the time of this evaluation. She followed instructions without difficulty.

Assessment

Dysphagia with risk for aspiration.

Plan

1. Maximize efficiency and safety of swallow through exercises to strengthen oral-motor and laryngeal musculature and establishment of swallowing precautions. Train nursing staff and family to cue Ms. Muñoz to utilize chin tucks and use double swallow and cough to clear the airway when needed when swallowing liquids.
2. Continue management of hearing at the Katze Clinic.

_____
Name, CCC-SLP; State Lic #, SLP
Speech–Language Pathologist

Samples of Integrated Reports

Samples of integrated team reports are provided in this appendix. The first is an example of a team report about a child referred to a cleft palate, craniofacial team based on the child's hypernasal speech production. The second report is an example of an augmentative communication (AC) evaluation, which is being submitted as a request to Medicaid for funds to purchase an AC device.

Sample 1: Integrated Report for Cleft Palate

Re: Smith, Roy

Sex: Male

Birthdate: 9-25-94

Parents: J.D. and Susan Smith

Address: Route #1, Dallas, TX

Telephone:

Date of Evaluation: July 15, 1999

Roy was first evaluated in this Center on June 13, 1999. At that time, he had a bifid uvula and possibly a submucous cleft palate. Velopharyngeal closure needed to be assessed because the child was noticeably hypernasal during speech production. Roy's half brother, James, has a cleft palate and also is being followed at this Center. Results of an audiometric test on June 13 indicated the presence of a slight to mild bilateral conductive hearing loss. The child was subsequently referred to ENT and is being followed there. He returns to ENT today for re-examination.

Summary of Findings

Plastic Surgery: The uvula is bifid and there is a submucous cleft of the velum. Velar motion is good. Speech is poor. (Dr. Baker)

As I view it, velar motion did not seem adequate. I would describe this as a "lazy palate." (Dr. Green)

Orthodontia: Roy presents early mixed dentition. Occlusal and jaw development are well within acceptable limits. (Dr. Lake)

Speech–Language Pathology: Mother reports that Roy has had recent ear infections. As previously noted, he presents a bifid uvula and submucous cleft palate. Videonasoendo-

scopic assessment reveals some observable lateral pharyngeal wall movement during phonation. Speech is moderately hypernasal. Fricatives are distorted. During conversation his receptive skills appear normal for his age. Expressively he used one- and two-word responses and appeared hesitant to converse with examiners. (Dr. Floyd)

Roy's speech is severely hypernasal and his articulation is poor. Velar length is good but mobility appears limited. Review of the videonasoendoscopic findings indicate that velopharyngeal closure is not effected. A submucous cleft is evident and there is a bony defect in the posterior part of the hard palate. (Dr. West)

Audiology: Roy failed an audiometric screening test. (Dr. Verner)

Summary of Recommendations

1. Complete hearing evaluation.

2. Refer for a complete speech and language evaluation.

3. Review by the entire team of the endoscopic study of velopharyngeal valving in connected speech.

4. If the team agrees, then surgery will be indicated. A Wardall pushback repair of submucous cleft, and superiorly based posterior pharyngeal flap (in one operation) are suggested.

5. Recall in 3 months (or as soon as recommendation #2 has been completed).

6. If middle ear problems persist, bilateral myringotomies with tubes may need to be coordinated with any future surgery.

Coordinator, Cleft Palate Center

Sample 2: Augmentative Communication Team Evaluation Report

Assistive Technology Center

Augmentative Communication Evaluation

Client's Name: Don Brown

Date of Birth: 6-10-41

Date of Evaluation: 7-6-98

Age: 57 years

Background Information

Mr. Brown was referred for an augmentative communication evaluation by the Westwood Speech and Hearing Clinic due to concerns about his inability to speak. Mr. Brown was initially referred to the Westwood Clinic by his physician in February 1996 for a speech and language evaluation. He suffered a CVA involving the left middle cerebral artery in May 1995, which resulted in right hemiplegia and aphasia. Findings from the first evaluation indicated that Mr. Brown was nonverbal, unable to voice, and experiencing swallowing difficulties. Auditory comprehension appeared adequate for daily living activities. A subsequent evaluation through the ENT clinic at Middleburg Medical Center in March 1995 revealed paresis of the right vocal fold and only a slight wave motion of the left vocal fold. The epiglottis did not move and Mr. Brown was unable to perform oral motor and facial movements. Diagnosis was apparent superior laryngeal nerve palsy and possible IXth nerve palsy as a result of the CVA. An audiological evaluation indicated hearing within normal limits. Vision was normal with corrective lenses. Mr. Brown was enrolled in speech treatment in March 1996 with goals to improve swallowing and oral motor function so that an electrolarynx could be used as a speech prosthesis. After a year of treatment with reportedly little improvement, these goals were abandoned and efforts to teach Mr. Brown sign language were initiated. However, this communication method was also terminated when little progress was made after 6 months. Although Mr. Brown was able to use a few gestures, his ability to sign or write was limited by what appeared to be a significant limb apraxia. For the last several months, treatment efforts have focused on using a picture communication system. Mr. Brown has been using a looseleaf notebook with line-drawn symbols arranged by category (food, clothing, feelings, health, etc.) to indicate basic needs.

Mr. Brown is a high school graduate and owned a small repair shop for several years before his CVA. After a brief stay at a nursing home, he was discharged to his mother's home where he now resides. He is divorced with three grown children who live out of state. Mr. Brown is ambulatory and is able to independently perform activities of daily living; however, he has not been able to continue employment due to his ongoing medical problems. He receives monthly disability benefits from Social Security, but has no other source of income. Mr. Brown has medical appointments at Middleburg Medical Center on a regular basis, but cannot communicate with his doctors. This is particularly distressing when he is not feeling well or in case of an emergency. In addition, Mr. Brown's ability to participate in activities with his family and friends is significantly impaired by his lack of speech and voice. He has reportedly indicated through picture symbols his frustration at not being able to communicate and has expressed a strong desire for obtaining an augmentative communication device with voice output.

Evaluation Questions

What are Mr. Brown's current motor, perceptual, and speech and language skills? Is he a candidate for a dedicated communication device? If so, which augmentative communication device would be most appropriate?

Assessment Method

Review of Records

Motor-Free Visual Perception Test–Revised

Test of Nonverbal Intelligence (TONI–2)

Peabody Picture Vocabulary Test–Third Edition (PPVT–III)

Boston Diagnostic Aphasia Test

Pyramids and Palm Trees Test

Informal Communication Sample

Oral Peripheral Examination

Clinical Observations

Family Interview

Hearing Screening

Evaluation Results

Motor and Positioning

Mr. Brown was ambulatory. Strength and range of motion were equal bilaterally and within functional limits. Balance and coordination in standing were functional when his hands were free for protective extension or for assistance with support. Mr. Brown was able to hold a pencil in his right hand and laboriously sign his name. He was also able to use his right index finger to accurately point to small pictures and symbols. A bilateral hand tremor was noted during the evaluation and was more significant on the left than the right. Mr. Brown did not use his left hand for stabilizing his paper as he wrote. He had difficulty with diadochokinetic movements and was unable to imitate hand patterns and movements that would be necessary for using an unaided communication system.

Perceptual Skills

Visually, Mr. Brown was able to track a visual stimulus horizontally across the midline. Tracking from midline to the left was more uncoordinated than right to midline. Functionally, he was able to identify symbols in all quadrants of the visual field suggesting no visual field deficits which would interfere with functional use of a communication device. The *Motor-Free Visual Perceptual Test* assesses five areas of visual perception in random order. Mr. Brown was required to point to the correct response figure which matched the stimulus figure. His visual perception was below normal limits, particularly in the areas of position in space and visual closure. This would contribute to his significant difficulty in producing a complete phrase or sentence through the written mode.

Cognitive Status

The TONI–2 was administered to estimate Mr. Brown's nonverbal cognitive skills. Although this test only requires a pointing response and is independent of speech and language skills, it does require adequate visual-perceptual skills. Since Mr. Brown also has difficulty in this area (see previous paragraph), his score may be an underestimate of his cognitive ability. With a mean of 100 and a standard deviation of 15, Mr. Brown's standard score of 84 was approximately one standard deviation below the mean for his chronological age. He obtained a percentile rank of 14. Informal observation indicated cognitive ability to be adequate for functional communication. Over the course of speech treatment, Mr. Brown has reportedly learned new tasks quickly and usually wins any dominoes game. During the evaluation, he was able to use an augmentative communication device with a dynamic display after just one demonstration. Results from previous testing indicated a seventh-grade reading level and an ability to do simple addition and subtraction problems.

Language Skills

Single-word receptive vocabulary was assessed with the PPVT–III. Mr. Brown earned a standard score of 78 (mean: 100; standard deviation: 15); a percentile rank of 7; and an age equivalency score of 14 years, 3 months. Several subtests from the *Boston Diagnostic Aphasia Test* were given to measure auditory comprehension, reading comprehension, and writing.

The writing subtest of the *Boston Diagnostic Aphasia Test* was discontinued because of Mr. Brown's inability to complete tasks such as "Spelling to Dictation." Although he was able to block print letters and numbers which were dictated, he could not spell words or write words spontaneously. Writing efforts were also slow and laborious. Other subtest scores indicated good auditory and reading comprehension for words, phrases, and sentences.

The *Pyramids and Palm Trees Test* is used to assess an individual's ability to access detailed semantic representations from words or pictures. The picture form was used with Mr. Brown. He had a total correct score of 48 out of a possible 52, a score of 92% correct. This score indicates adequate understanding of concrete picture associations.

Throughout the current evaluation, Mr. Brown followed complex directions correctly. He responded to questions by nodding or shaking his head, although he had some difficulty initiating lateral head movement to indicate "no." He also attempted to indicate numbers by showing the correct number

of fingers, but had difficulty with these movements as well. He did not spontaneously use other gestures. His grandson reported that Mr. Brown will sometimes bring his picture notebook to a member of the family and point to a symbol for what he wants. During part of the evaluation, Mr. Brown was given an augmentative communication device (Macaw, from Zygo) with picture symbols and vocabulary for playing dominoes. He quickly learned the line-drawn symbols and used them appropriately during several games. Although facial affect was quite flat and Mr. Brown only rarely smiled, he did indicate his enjoyment of the game by pointing to the symbol for "let's play again."

Speech/Oral-Motor Skills

Informal assessment of swallowing and voice revealed an inability to produce voice or an adequate air stream as well as difficulty with saliva control. Mr. Brown kept a handkerchief in his pocket, which he used frequently to wipe his mouth. According to his family, he continues to have significant difficulty managing liquids and certain foods. When asked to imitate oral motor movements performed by the examiner, he was able to open and close his mouth, but could not perform other tasks such as protruding/retracting tongue, puckering lips, and so on. As reported earlier, extensive treatment to improve swallowing and oral motor skills was unsuccessful as were attempts at using an electrolarynx. Mr. Brown could not sequence speech sounds into words and phrases which is necessary for using this type of speech prosthesis successfully.

Hearing Screening

Mr. Brown responded to pure tone stimuli presented at screening levels in both ears.

Communication Needs Inventory

Mr. Brown's frequent communication partners include family members, friends, medical personnel, therapists, receptionists, and store clerks. In addition to being able to express his medical needs and discuss his medical condition with medical personnel, Mr. Brown needs to be able to converse with both family and friends. His need for written communication is limited at this time since he is not employed and can write his name when he is required to do so. However, he may eventually wish to communicate through letters to his grandson. Although Mr. Brown spends most of his time at home, he goes to speech treatment weekly and to the hospital for frequent medical checkups. He would also like to attend church and some social functions if he had a way to communicate with others. His outings are also limited due to a lack of transportation. Mr. Brown would like to have his own personal car in order to be more independent and has expressed a desire to work again. This seems to be a reasonable goal. If this occurs, then the number of communication environments and communication partners would likely expand. For now, vocabulary and message needs would include at least the following categories: Medical, food and drink, family members, clothing, social phrases, games (e.g., dominoes and cards), places, and personal history.

Required Features of AAC Device

From the evaluation data and treatment notes, it was determined that Mr. Brown would access a communication device through the direct selection method of touching the screen or keys with his finger. The device would need to provide speech/voice output, including an alarm or other loud signaling mechanism since the absence of speech or voice is Mr. Brown's most significant deficit. Although written communication needs are limited at this time, a device which provides this option would assure that all future needs would be met with the purchase of this device. Any selected device should have the capability of enlarging symbols and print to meet changing visual needs; allow for expanding vocabulary and message needs; provide ways to increase the rate of message production as well as correctability of messages; and be "user friendly" in terms of programming so that Mr. Brown can achieve complete independence in using this device.

Since Mr. Brown is ambulatory, the device should also be lightweight and portable. He will need a way to transport the device from place to place as well as a means of supporting it as he uses it. The device will need to be mounted on a desk or table top when he is sitting and using it at home. For walking, he will require a strap or other carrying device which supports the device at waist level by suspending it from the shoulders. This method would allow Mr. Brown's arms and hands to be free for support and protective extension at the same time that the device is readily available for communication.

AAC Devices Considered

Mr. Brown was given the opportunity to use a variety of different augmentative communication devices over the course of several months, including the Parrot and Macaw from Zygo; the MessageMate and Finger Foniks from Words+; and the DynaVox from Sentient Systems. Of these, the two devices from Words+ were ruled out after a trial period due to Mr. Brown's difficulty with spelling. Other small portable devices such as the Canon Communicator and the Lightwriter were also ruled out for the same reason; they use a keyboard and require the user to be a quick and accurate speller. At that point it was determined that Mr. Brown would need a picture/symbol based system. Although Mr. Brown could easily use the Parrot and Macaw, these devices are limited to a small set of messages. This type of device would not meet the needs of someone of Mr. Brown's age, language ability, and cognitive status. The DynaVox meets all of the communication needs, but is too heavy to be a practical consideration for an ambulatory person. However, the DynaMyte (also from Sentient Systems) is small and lightweight. It can easily be carried by hand or by shoulder strap. The DynaMyte has many of the same features as the DynaVox including a dynamic display (similar to a computer screen), which removes the cognitive and memory demands of a static display; the ability to store thousands of preprogrammed messages for rapid communication; the ability to also create novel messages; rechargeable battery; and customized voice.

The DynaMyte is the most cost-effective alternative for meeting Mr. Brown's communication needs. First, through the expanded memory and capacity for written output as well as speech, it would meet all future needs if Mr. Brown's skills improve or the number of communication partners and environments increases. At the same time, this device can be reduced in sophistication and has alternative access capability if his medical condition should deteriorate. By having this type of speech prosthesis, costly medical problems may actually be prevented or at least reduced since Mr. Brown would be able to actively participate in his medical care. Finally, the DynaMyte would help Mr. Brown achieve more independence since he would no longer have to rely on others to "talk" for him and might eventually help him obtain employment.

Mr. Brown has been working in speech treatment with a DynaVox (which belongs to the speech clinic) for approximately a month and has become proficient at using it to participate in treatment activities. He fully understands the organization of the device in categories or "pages" and how to quickly move from one page to another. Even though his visual scanning ability has not always been efficient, this has reportedly become less of an issue as he has learned the location of each symbol. He also performed well when given an opportunity to try the DynaMyte in a session with the vendor. During this session, Mr. Brown expressed a preference for the DynaMyte because of its size and weight and the color display, which appeared to better meet his visual and perceptual needs.

Summary

Mr. Brown is a 57-year-old male who has a primary communication diagnosis of aphasia and a secondary diagnosis of apraxia and dysphagia as the result of a CVA involving the middle cerebral artery in May 1995. A medical evaluation in 1996 also revealed paresis of the right vocal fold and suspected damage to the superior laryngeal nerve. Mr. Brown has been receiving speech treatment services for the past 2 years. Efforts to regain speech and adequate oral motor function have not been successful and attempts at teaching other communication methods such as use of an electrolarynx or gesture and writing system have also failed due to his severe verbal and limb apraxia. At this time, Mr. Brown still cannot speak or vocalize; however, his auditory comprehension and cognitive status are good. This results in significant unmet communication needs and puts him at increased risk medically. It also restricts Mr. Brown's ability to become more independent, which he has expressed a desire to be and could be with an effective and efficient means to communicate with others.

Recommendations

After numerous trials with other devices as well as a successful trial period with the requested device, we are recommending the DynaMyte from Sentient Systems Technology because it best meets Mr. Brown's current and future communication needs as well as his need for portability and access. Mr. Brown also expressed a preference for this device and was eager to learn how to use it, which is important because of the amount of commitment the training will require. This training will be provided by both the manufacturing representative and by the augmentative communication specialist working with Mr.

Brown in his speech treatment program. In addition to the device itself, we are also recommending a carrying case to increase portability and durability.

It is also recommended that Mr. Brown continue to have his looseleaf communication notebook available as a backup method of communication in case the battery of the DynaMyte needs charging or the device is in need of repair, and that he use body gestures, eye contact, and facial expressions as much as possible for communication. If Mr. Brown cannot provide his own transportation to activities in the community, then other resources should be investigated such as medical transportation.

Treatment Plan and Follow-Up

The long-term goal of treatment is for Mr. Brown to use the DynaMyte independently and spontaneously as a speech prosthesis. This would include learning how to program the device independently as well. Speech treatment services would be discontinued when this goal is met. Other possible outcomes of treatment would be that Mr. Brown could live independently, participate more fully in society, and perhaps once again be employed if his health continues to improve. Short-term goals

would include using the device to respond to questions; using prestored messages to greet, request, comment, ask questions, etc. (gradually moving from clinician prompting to spontaneous use); using the device to create novel messages (with prompting, then spontaneously); using word prediction and abbreviations to speed up communication; and learning programming and troubleshooting when breakdowns occur. These goals should be accomplished within a year of Mr. Brown's receiving his device. Periodic follow-up by the manufacturing representative and augmentative communication specialist will be provided. In addition, Sentient Systems provides technical support through a toll free number and offers new product information and learning opportunities on an ongoing basis.

Name, CCC-SLP; State Lic #, SLP
Speech–Language Pathologist

Name, LOTR, State Lic #
Occupational Therapist

Samples of Treatment Plans and Progress Reports

The first sample of a treatment plan and progress report concerns the 69-year-old man with aphasia described in Appendix A, Report 10. The second sample concerns the same elderly client with dysphagia described in Appendix A, Report 11, and in the sixth example of a Problem Oriented Report in Appendix B. These are written in an abbreviated style similar to that used in acute care and rehabilitation hospitals and nursing homes.

Sample 1

Client in Report 10, Appendix A

Mr. Smith, age 69 years

Medical Diagnosis: Aphasia following CVA

Frequency of Treatment: Daily sessions for 4 weeks

Problem: Aphasia with cognitive and linguistic deficits

Plan of Treatment: Individual treatment with SLP; use of visual, verbal, and tactile activities; use of external aids to increase orientation (such as a memory book); staff, patient, and family education; and a weekly meeting of the rehabilitation team.

Functional Goals

Increase functional communication and comprehension of oral and written language to improve the level of his safety in the home environment.

Long Term

Independent living in the home environment.

Short Term

1. Mr. Smith will increase orientation in time and space for his current environment with 80% accuracy in the clinical setting.
2. He will increase his level of reasoning and problem-solving skills to 80% accuracy in the clinical setting.
3. He will improve word finding abilities in order to increase functional communication skills by 80% in the clinical setting.
4. He will improve reading comprehension of 2 to 3 sentences to 80% accuracy.
5. He will identify main idea/topic of auditorily presented reading passage or conversation at 80% accuracy.

Functional Abilities at Outset of Treatment (9/22/1999)	At End of Treatment (10/20/1999)
1. Confused orientation when interacting with more than one person at a time with difficulty in concentration and attention	Well oriented with two people in room with 80% accuracy
2. Reasoning and problem-solving skills at 60% accuracy	75% accuracy
3. Word finding abilities 50% of the time	25% of the time
4. Reading comprehension in short passages at 60% accuracy	Comprehension of 2- to 3-word reading passages at 75% accuracy
5. Ability to identify main topic/idea of auditorily presented reading passage or conversation was limited by attention and concentration difficulties	Identified main topic: Auditorily: 85%; Reading: 80%; Conversation: 90%

Recommendations

Schedule an additional session to provide the patient and family with specific activities to improve orientation, reading, comprehension, and functional communication in the home environment. A follow-up examination should be done in 6 months.

Name, CCC-SLP; State Lic #, SLP
Speech–Language Pathologist

Sample 2

Client in Report 11, Appendix A

Ms. Muñoz, age 86 years

Medical Diagnosis: Pneumonia accompanied by dysphagia; Hearing loss

Frequency of Treatment: 3 times a week for 4 weeks (2/8 through 3/8/2000)

Problem: Risk of aspiration

Plan of Treatment: Oral motor/laryngeal strengthening exercises; establish swallowing precautions program. Ms. Muñoz should wear her hearing aids during all treatment sessions.

Functional Goals

Long Term

Maximize efficiency and safety of swallow.

Short Term

1. Ms. Muñoz will perform oral motor exercises with 70% accuracy within 3 weeks.
2. She will perform laryngeal strengthening exercises with 60% accuracy within 3 weeks.
3. She will perform chin tucks 100% of the time when drinking liquids within 3 weeks.
4. She will be cued to use double swallows as needed by nursing staff, family, and speech–language pathologist for 3 weeks.
5. She will cough/clear after liquid presentations as needed within 3 weeks.
6. She will wear her hearing aids 100% of the time while she is awake.

Functional Abilities at Outset of Treatment (2/8/2000)	At End of Treatment (3/3/2000)
1. Completes oral-motor exercises with 50% accuracy	75% (25% increase)
2. Correctly does laryngeal, pushing, and sucking exercises with 50% accuracy	70% (20% increase)
3. Utilizes appropriately the chin tuck technique as needed without cuing (At outset used chin tuck 80%)	100% (20% increase)
4. Uses double swallow and cough/clear technique when a wet voice is present following swallowing clear liquids	Still needs cuing
5. Requires reminding to wear hearing aids 20% of the time	0% (20% increase)

Recommendations

Conduct one more session to train nursing staff, patient, and family to cue and respond to cues to utilize chin tucks, double swallows, cough/clear as needed during swallowing liquids, and assist with hearing aid use.

Name, CCC-SLP; State Lic #, SLP
Speech–Language Pathologist

Samples of Individualized Education Programs (IEPs)

The first IEP sample is for the 4-year-old child with a phonological disorder presented in Report 3 of Appendix A. The second sample is for the preschool-aged child with a resonance voice disorder presented in Report 6 of Appendix A.

 Sample 1

Client in Report 3, Appendix A

Identifying Information: David, age 4 years, 5 months
Grade: Preschool
Language: English

Present Level of Performance

Language

Scores on subtests of the *Test of Language Development–Primary: Third Edition* that measure understanding and meaningful use of spoken words, grammar, and word discrimination were normal for his age.

Phonological

Phonological error patterns were assessed using Hodson's *Assessment of Phonological Processes*. Error patterns included numerous sound substitutions and occasional sound omissions. Omissions included reduction of consonant blends (e.g., "back" for *black*) and sound substitutions included stopping of fricatives in the word initial position (e.g, "pish" for *fish*), deaffrication of affricates in the word final position (e.g., "wat" for *watch*), and replacement of liquids with glides (e.g, "wing" for *ring*). He uses a broad phonetic inventory of speech sounds, though not always correctly, including the stop phonemes p, b, k, g; fricatives s and sh; and nasals m, n, and ng. He was stimulable with auditory and visual cues in producing correctly various consonant blends, fricatives, and affricates.

Connected Speech

David's connected speech is judged to be about 50% intelligible. With careful listening in a known context, his speech intelligibility is increased to about 75%. He used five- and six-word utterances mingled occasionally with complex sentences containing as many as 10 words. Semantics, syntax, and pragmatic skills were appropriate for his age.

Hearing, Oral Structure and Function, Fluency, and Voice

Normal based on screenings.

Educational Impact

It is difficult for David's teachers and peers to understand his speech, particularly when they are unaware of the context or subject matter of his utterances. He has strong underlying language skills including well-organized sentence structure. Thus, his potential for academic achievement is excellent but is being inhibited by his lack of ability to get his ideas across to listeners efficiently.

Objectives

Long-Term Objectives

David's speech intelligibility will be increased to 100% by the end of the school year.

Short-Term Objectives

Correct response rates will be charted for each objective at least once each week.

1. David will produce the following correctly in drilled responses to examiner productions and pictures in 8 out of 10 consecutive single words:

   consonant–s blends   Date Accomplished: _____

   consonant–l blends   Date Accomplished: _____

   fricatives (s, sh, f, v)   Date Accomplished: _____

2. David will produce the following correctly in drilled responses to examiner productions and pictures in 8 out of 10 consecutive single words:

   liquids   Date Accomplished: _____

3. David will produce s and l blends in three- and four-word phrases in response to drills using objects and pictures.

   Date Accomplished: _____

4. David will produce fricatives s, sh, f, and v in three- and four-word phrases in response to drills using objects and pictures.

Date Accomplished: _____

5. David will produce consonant–s and consonant–l blends in clinician monitored conversations in varied settings.

Date Accomplished: _____

6. David will produce fricatives in clinician-monitored conversations in varied settings.

Date Accomplished: _____

7. David will produce liquids in three- and four-word phrases in response to drills using objects and pictures.

Date Accomplished: _____

8. David will use consonant blends, fricatives, and liquids in spontaneous speech in varied settings.

Date Accomplished: _____

Treatment Schedule

David will be seen for individual treatment three times each week for 30-minute sessions.

A 30-minute consult by the speech–language pathologist with the teacher targeting techniques to facilitate generalization of David's corrected speech patterns in the classroom setting will be held each week.

Regular Education Program

David attends half-day preschool 4 hours a day, 20 hours per week; he will attend regular preschool education class 18.5 hours a week (1.5 hours spent in speech treatment).

Treatment Schedule

Date of IEP Meeting: 9/15/1999

Date Treatment Begins: 9/17/1999

Date Treatment Ends: 5/22/2000

Rationale for Special Education Services

Conversational speech is 50% intelligible. Speech needs cannot be met in a regular education classroom.

Professionals Providing the Services

School Speech–Language Pathologist

Classroom Teacher: In collaboration with the speech-language pathologist

_____
(Parents, SLP, Classroom Teacher)

 Sample 2

Client in Report 6, Appendix A

Identifying Information: Homer, age 4 years, 9 months

Grade: Preschool

Language: English

Present Level of Performance

Language

Receptive One-Word Picture Vocabulary Test: He scored 96, age equivalent of 4 years, 7 months.

Structured Photographic Expressive Language Test–II (SPELT–II), a standardized measure for production of specific morphological and syntactical structure: He scored 5 (mean score for a child his chronological age is 22.39).

Oral Language Imitation Sentence Test–Stage III: His mean length of imitative utterance was 5.2.

He imitated most linguistic structures but with some reduction of sentence length.

Based on an analysis of a spontaneous language sample, Homer's mean length of utterance was 3.25. He used present progressive verbs (e.g., *smiling*) and prepositions (e.g.,

in, on, under), but did not use past tense verbs in the sample.

Articulation

Iowa Pressure Articulation Test, a subtest of the *Templin–Darley Tests of Articulation* that assesses the adequacy of oral pressure for speech sound production and thus, inferentially, the adequacy of velopharyngeal closure during speech. Productions included the following errors: weak pressure consonants and substitution of glottal stops.

On the *Weighted Values for Speech Symptoms Associated with VPI*, which is based on symptoms heard or seen during speech, his scores was 12. A score of 7 or above suggests velopharyngeal incompetency.

Speech Sample

Spontaneous speech characterized by nasal emission, hypernasality, nasal grimacing, hoarseness, breathiness, and glottal stop substitutions.

Instrumental Assessment

Difference in mean scores for nonnasal and nasal reading on the Nasometer was 9.41, which is not a significant difference, implying the presence of hypernasality during speech.

Oral Structure and Function

Bifid uvula, hypertrophied palatine tonsils, bony deficiency on posterior margin of hard palate.

Hearing

Passed hearing screening; history of otitis media and PE tubes in both ears. The PE tube in the right eardrum appears to be coming out; normal middle ear pressure and function were found in the left ear where PE tube is intact.

Voice

Dysphonia; voice is judged hoarse and rough.

Fluency

Normal

Educational Impact

It is difficult for Homer's preschool teachers and peers to understand his hoarse and hypernasal speech. Expressively he does not use the length and complexity of sentences in conversation expected of a child his age.

Objectives

Long-Term Objectives (End of the school year)

1. With a team approach, Homer's phonatory hoarseness will be eliminated as judged by the educational and medical team.

2. With a team approach, Homer's hypernasal resonance will be reduced significantly according to Nasometer ratings.

3. Homer's use of syntactical and morphological structures will be within normal limits for a child his age as measured by the SPELT–II.

Short-Term Objectives

1. Homer will have been evaluated by the school-based voice team to determine the status of previously identified vocal fold nodules and the status of his velopharyngeal mechanism.

    Date Accomplished: _____

2. Homer will be aware of three vocal abuses and will practice decreasing them in the clinical setting. The three abuses will be listed and progress on implementing solutions will be recorded and provided to the parents.

    Date Accomplished: _____

3. Homer will be aware of five (including the three from Objective 1) vocal abuses and will practice decreasing them in the clinical and the classroom settings.

    Date Accomplished: _____

4. The family will follow up on recommendations by the voice team and reports of findings will be available to the educational team including the parents.

    Date Accomplished: _____

5. Homer's parents and teachers will consistently reinforce Homer for reducing previously identified vocal abuses. Their reports of Homer's progress will be documented in treatment files.

6. During the final 6 weeks evaluation period, Homer's velopharyngeal function and condition of his vocal folds will be reevaluated by the voice team with findings shared with the educational team including the parents.

    Date Accomplished: _____

7. Homer will reduce the number of vocal abuses reported by teachers and parents by 10%.

    Date Accomplished: _____

8. Homer will use complete grammatically correct sentences during conversation. He will make no more than 2 errors during 5 minutes of conversation.

    Date Accomplished: _____

9. Homer will use grammatically complete sentences during conversation commensurate with his age level with no more than one error per treatment session.

    Date Accomplished: _____

Treatment Schedule

Homer will be seen for small group treatment 3 times each week for 30 minutes and 1 time a week individually for 30 minutes. A 15-minute consult by the speech–language pathologist with the teacher in the classroom to identify and develop strategies for reducing vocal abuses in the classroom.

Regular Education Program

Homer attends half-day preschool 4 hours a day, 20 hours per week. He will attend regular preschool education class 18.5 hours a week (1.5 hours spent in speech treatment).

Treatment Schedule

Date of IEP Meeting: 9/8/2000
Date Treatment Begins: 9/13/2000
Date Treatment Ends: 5/22/2001

Rationale for Special Education Services

Homer presents delayed expressive language skills with errors in syntax and morphology and reduced speech intelligibility due to hypernasal speech. His language and speech needs cannot be met in the regular education classroom.

Professionals Providing the Services

Speech–Language Pathologist

Classroom Teacher: In collaboration with the Speech–Language Pathologist

Voice Team: ENT Physician, Voice Specialist Speech–Language Pathologist

Signatures:

_____

(Parents, SLP, Teacher, Voice Team Members)

Sample of an Individualized Family Service Plan (IFSP)

The IFSP sample is for the preschool-aged child with a delay in language acquisition described in Report 7 of Appendix A.

 Sample

Client in Report 7, Appendix A

Identifying Information: Karen, age 20 months
Language in Home: English

History

Karen reached motor milestones normally. Her mother reports she has no spoken words at this time. She hears some sounds, but does not demonstrate consistent comprehension of speech. She has a history of ear infections prior to insertion of ventilating tubes on June 10, 2001. She is seeing her otolaryngologist for regular visits every 3 to 4 months.

Present Level of Performance

Examination

Last of three hearing evaluations completed on November 8, 1999. Responses to warbled tone stimuli were consistent at 45 to 50 dBHL for air conduction. However, Karen responded several times to pure tones presented at 20 to 25 dBHL. Speech awareness was established at 25 dBHL. Immittance measurements revealed a normal trace for the left ear and functioning ventilation tube or perforated eardrum in the right ear. Otoscopic inspection revealed a ventilation tube in the right tympanic membrane and the left eardrum appeared intact. Bone conduction was not attempted because she would not tolerate the bone conduction oscillator.

Karen imitated the examiner during play activity and used gestures and vocalizations to ask for specific toys that were out of her reach. She resisted eye contact with the examiner and was easily distracted. She imitated motor activities during play but would not imitate the examiner's repetitive syllables or monosyllabic words.

Family

The family has a history of following up on all recommendations. They are well read about hearing loss.

Intervention Goals (Measurement of Progress)

1. Evaluate the child's hearing using brainstem audiometrics. Results will be provided in report form and explained to the educational team including the parents.

2. Continue follow-up medical assessments by the otolaryngologist. The parents will provide the educational team with reports (written or verbal) of each visit. Information will be placed in the child's file.

3. Schedule a speech and language evaluation with a school speech-language pathologist on the child's educational team. The results of that examination will be provided in written form and the speech–language pathologist will report findings at the next meeting of the educational team.

4. The school speech–language pathologist will make monthly 1-hour visits to the child's home to provide parents with strategies for facilitating speech and language development in the home environment. The parents will document the child's speech attempts in a diary for the speech-language pathologist to review at each visit.

Treatment Schedule

Date Treatment Begins: 10/4/2001
Evaluation Scheduled: 10/4/2001
First Monthly Visit: 10/11/2001
Date Treatment Ends: 6/14/2002

Treatment Team

Educational Audiologist (Case Manager)
Speech-Language Pathologist
Signatures:

_____
Educational Audiologist

_____
Speech–Language Pathologist

References

American Psychological Association. (1994). *Publication manual of the American Psychological Association*. Washington, DC: Author.

American Speech-Language-Hearing Association. (1979). Guidelines for nonsexist language in the journals of ASHA. *Asha, 21*(11), 973–976.

American Speech-Language-Hearing Association. (1989). *Consumer satisfaction measure*. Rockville, MD: Author.

American Speech-Language-Hearing Association. (1990). Code of ethics of the American Speech-Language-Hearing Association. *Asha, 32*(3), 91–92.

American Speech-Language-Hearing Association. (1991–1992). The publication process: A guide for authors. *National Student Speech-Language-Hearing Association Journal 19*, 138–142.

American Speech-Language-Hearing Association. (1992, March). Statement of practices and procedures: Ethical practice board. *Asha, 34*(Suppl. 13), 3–5.

American Speech-Language-Hearing Association. (1993). Guidelines for gender equality in language use. *Asha, 35*(Suppl. 10), 42–46.

American Speech-Language-Hearing Association. (1994a). Code of ethics. *Asha, 36*(Suppl. 13), 1–2.

American Speech-Language-Hearing Association. (1994b, March). Conflicts of professional interest. *Asha, 36* (Suppl. 13), 7–8.

American Speech-Language-Hearing Association. (1995a). *American Professional Services Board Standards and Accreditation Manual*. Rockville, MD: Author.

American Speech-Language-Hearing Association. (1995b). *National treatment outcome data collection project: User's guide phase 1–Group 1*. Rockville, MD: Author.

American Speech-Language-Hearing Association. (1995c). Treatment outcome: Task force update. *Asha, 37*(6/7), 26.

American-Speech-Language-Hearing-Association. (1995d). *User's guide phase I: Group II Healthcare*. Rockville, MD: Author.

American Speech-Language-Hearing Association. (1996a). *National treatment outcome data collection project: National report cards numbers 1–8 adults in health care settings*. Rockville, MD: Author.

American Speech-Language-Hearing Association. (1996b). Scope of practice in audiology. *Asha, 38*(Suppl. 16), 12–15.

American Speech-Language-Hearing Association. (1996c). Scope of practice in speech–language pathology. *Asha, 38*(Suppl. 16), 16–20.

American Speech-Language-Hearing Association. (1996d). *User's guide phase I: Group III*. Rockville, MD: Author.

American Speech-Language-Hearing Association. (1997a). *Characteristics of State Licensure Laws*. Rockville, MD: Author.

American Speech-Language-Hearing Association. (1997b). *Preferred practice patterns for the profession of audiology*. Rockville, MD: Author.

American Speech-Language-Hearing Association. (1997c). *Preferred practice patterns for the profession of speech–language pathology*. Rockville, MD: Author.

American Speech-Language-Hearing Association. (1997d). Treatment outcomes in voice: Client/caregiver rating questionnaire. *ASHA Special Interests Division: Voice and Voice Disorders, 7*(1), 181.

American Speech-Language-Hearing Association. (1998a). *Council on academic accreditation*. Rockville, MD: Author.

American Speech-Language-Hearing Association. (1998b). *Journal clubs*. Rockville, MD: Author.

American Speech-Language-Hearing Association. (1998c). *Manuscript checklist*. Rockville, MD: Author.

American Speech-Language-Hearing Association. (1998d). *National outcomes measurement system: Annual report—adults*. Rockville, MD: Author.

American Speech-Language-Hearing Association. (1999a). *ASHA code of ethics*. Rockville, MD: Author.

American Speech-Language-Hearing Association. (1999b). *For life after your graduate school*. Rockville, MD: Author.

American Speech-Language-Hearing Association. (1999c). *National outcomes measurement system: Annual report—acute rehabilitation*. Rockville, MD: Author.

American Speech-Language-Hearing Association. (1999d). *National outcomes measurement system: Annual report—rehabilitation hospitals*. Rockville, MD: Author.

American Speech-Language-Hearing Association. (1999e). *National outcomes measurement system: Annual report—skilled nursing*. Rockville, MD: Author.

American Speech-Language-Hearing Association. (1999f). *Professional Services Board: Accreditation Manual*. Rockville, MD: Author.

Anderson, M. (1992). *Imposters in the temple*. New York: Simon and Schuster.

Anthony, R., & Roe, G. (1998). *Resumes for teachers*. Happase, NY: Barrons.

Apel, K. (1999). Checks and balances. Keeping the science in our profession. *Language, Speech, and Hearing Services in Schools, 30*(1), 98–107.

Bailar, J. C., & Mosteller, F. (1988). Guidelines for statistical reporting in articles for medical journals. *Annals of Internal Medicine 108*, 266–275.

Baldwin, C. D., Goldblum, R. M., Rassin, D. K., & Levie, H. G. (1994). Facilitating faculty development and research through critical review of grant proposals and articles. *Academic Medicine, 69*(1), 62–64.

Bangs, T. (1982). *Language and learning disorders of the preacademic child*. Englewood Cliffs, NJ: Prentice-Hall.

Bates, J. D., & Kromas, P. (1993). *Writing with precision: How to write so that you can't possibly be misunderstood*. Washington, DC: Acropolis.

Baxley, B., & Bowers, L. (1991–1992). Clinical report writing: The perceptions of supervisors and supervisees. *National Student Speech-Language-Hearing Association Journal, 19*, 35–40.

Beal, J., Lynch, M., & Moore, P. (1989). Views on research: Communicating nursing research: Another look at the use of poster sessions in undergraduate programs. *Nurse Educator, 14*(1), 8–10.

Beatty, R. H. (1984). *The resume kit*. New York: Wiley.

Benning, S. P., & Speer, S. C. (1993). Incorrect citations: A comparison of library literature with medical literature. *Bulletin of the Medical Library Association, 81*(1), 56–58.

Berger, A. A. (1993). *Improving writing skills*. Newbury Park, CA: Sage.

Berke, J. (1995). *Twenty questions for the writer.* New York: Harcourt, Brace.

Black, T. R. (1993). *Evaluating social science research.* Thousand Oaks, CA: Sage.

Blischak, D. M., & Ho, K. M. (2000). School-based augmentative and alternative communication evaluation reports. *Contemporary Issues in Communication Sciences and Disorders, 27,* 70–81.

Bloch, D. P. (1997). *How to write a winning resume.* Lincolnwood, IL: VGM Career Horizons.

Blum, J. (1984). *Guide to the whole writing process.* Boston: Houghton Mifflin College Division.

Boice, R. (1989). Procrastination, busyness and bingeing. *Behavior Research and Therapy, 27*(6), 605–611.

Booth, W. C., Colomb, G. G., & Williams, J. M. (1995). *The craft of research.* Chicago: The University of Chicago Press.

Bordens, K., & Abbott, B. (1988). *Research design and methods.* Mountain View, CA: Mayfield.

Bouchard, M., & Shane, H. (1977). Use of the problem-oriented medical records in the speech and hearing profession. *Asha, 19*(3), 157–159.

Boyce, B., & Banning, C. (1979). Data accuracy in citation studies. *Summer RQ, 18*(4), 349–350.

Braddom, C. (1990). A framework for writing and/or evaluating research papers. *American Journal of Physical Medicine and Rehabilitation, 69,* 333–335.

Bradley, S. G. (1995). Conflict of interest. In F. L. Meering (Ed.), *Scientific integrity* (pp. 161–187). Washington, DC: American Society for Microbiology.

Brecker, L. K. (1993, November 8). Ethics of HIVP: Fears, rights, and confidentiality. *Advance for Speech–Language Pathologists and Audiologists, 3*(23), 15, 24.

Burnard, P. (1992). *Writing for health professionals: A manual for writers.* London: Chapman and Hall.

Campbell, D. (1999a, August 30). Improving student outcomes. *Advance for Speech–Language Pathologists and Audiologists,* pp. 10–11.

Campbell, D. (1999b, September 20). Practicing under PPS: Innovative strategies to thrive in today's health care environment. *Advance for Speech–Language Pathologists and Audiologists, 9*(38), 9–10.

Campbell, D. (1999c, October 18). Outcomes in aphasia. *Advance for Speech–Language Pathologists and Audiologists,* pp. 6–9.

Carney, A. E., & Moeller, M. P. (1998). Treatment efficacy: Hearing loss in children. *Journal of Speech, Language, and Hearing Research 41*(1), 561–584.

Carter, T. (1986). Reflections on disability. *Breakthrough.* El Paso, TX: Opportunity Center for the Handicapped.

Centra, J. A. (1979). *Determining faculty effectiveness.* San Francisco: Jossey–Bass.

Chapey, R. (1977). Consumer satisfaction in speech–language pathology. *Asha, 19*(11), 829–833.

Cheney, T. (1983). *Getting the words right.* Cincinnati: Writer's Digest Books.

Chial, M. (1984). Evaluating microcomputer hardware. In A. Schwartz (Ed.), *Handbook of microcomputer applications in communication disorders* (pp. 79–125). San Diego: College Hill Press.

Chial, M. (1985). Scholarship as a process: A task analysis of thesis and dissertation research. *Seminars in Speech Language, 6*(1), 35–54.

Cho, M. K., & Bero, L. A. (1994). Instrument for assessing the quality of drug studies published in the medical literature. *Journal of the American Medical Association, 272*(2), 101–104.

Coelho, C. A., DeRuyter, F., & Stein, M. (1996). Treatment efficacy: Cognitive–communication disorders resulting from traumatic brain injury. *Journal of Speech and Hearing Research, 39*(5), S5–S17.

Coelho, R. J., & Saunders, J. L. (1997). Journal publication and peer review: Guidelines and standards for authors and reviewers. *Journal of Applied Rehabilitation Counseling, 28*(3), 18–22.

Cohen, C. (1984). Implementing microcomputer applications. In A. Schwartz (Ed.), *Handbook of microcomputer applications in communication disorders* (pp. 17–33). San Diego: College Hill Press.

Colditz, G. A., & Emerson, J. D. (1985). The statistical content of published medical research: Some implications for biomedical education. *Medical Education, 19,* 248–255.

Cole, P. A., & McNichol, J. G. (1997). *Tools for a successful job search.* Rockville, MD: American Speech-Language-Hearing Association.

Cone, J. D. (1993). *Dissertations and theses from start to finish.* Washington, DC: American Psychological Association.

Connell, P., & McReynolds, L. (1988). A clinical science approach to treatment. In N. Lass, L. McReynolds, J. Northern, & D. Yoder (Eds.), *Handbook of speech–language pathology and audiology* (pp. 1058–1073). Philadelphia: B. C. Decker.

Connell, P., & Thompson, C. (1986). Flexibility of single subject experimental designs: Part III. Using flexibility to design or modify experiments. *Journal of Speech and Hearing Disorders, 51*(3), 204–214.

Conture, E. G. (1996). Treatment efficiency: Stuttering. *Journal of Speech and Hearing Research, 39*(5), S18–S26.

Cooper, J., Hersch, S., & Trapp, J. (1988). Poster presentation: Technical considerations and format. *Hearsay,* pp. 28–29.

Cornett, B., & Chabon, S. (1988). *The clinical practice of speech–language pathology.* Columbus, OH: Merrill.

Coury, D. L. (1991). A guide to critical reading of the literature in behavioral and developmental pediatrics. *Developmental and Behavioral Pediatrics, 12*(6), 351–354.

Cox, R., & West, W. (1986). *Fundamentals of research for health professionals.* Rockville, MD: RAMSCO.

Coxford, L. M. (1987). *Resume writing made easy.* Scottsdale, AZ: Gorsuch Scarisbrick.

Crawford, H. (1998, September 21). Do's and don'ts of documentation. *ADVANCE for Speech–Language Pathologists and Audiologists, 8*(38), 7–8.

Creaghead, N. A. (1999). Evaluating language intervention approaches: Contrasting perspectives. *Language, Speech, and Hearing Services in Schools, 30,* 335–338.

Criscito, P. (1997). *Resumes in cyberspace.* Happase, NY: Barrons.

Culatta, R. A. (1984). Why articles don't get published in Asha. *Asha, 26*(3), 25–27.

Dalston, R. (1983). Computer–generated reports of speech and language evaluations. *Cleft Palate Journal, 20*(3), 227–237.

Dalton, R., & Dalton, M. (1990). *The student's guide to good writing.* New York: College Entrance Examination Board.

Darley, F. (1978a). The examination report. In F. Darley & D. Spriestersbach (Eds.), *Diagnostic methods in speech pathology* (pp. 400–405). New York: Harper & Row.

Darley, F. (1978b). A philosophy of appraisal and diagnosis. In F. Darley & D. Spriestersbach (Eds.), *Diagnostic methods in speech pathology* (pp. 1–36). New York: Harper & Row.

Davis, G., & Parker, C. (1979). *Writing the doctoral dissertation.* New York: Barron's Educational Series.

Davis, M. (1997). *Scientific papers and presentations.* New York: Academic Press.

Day, R. A. (1994). *How to write and publish a scientific paper.* Phoenix, AZ: Onyx Press.

DeLacey, G., Record, C., & Wade, J. (1985). How accurate are quotations and references in medical journals? *British Medical Journal, 291,* 884–886.

DePoy, E., & Gitlin, L. N. (1994). *Introduction to research.* St. Louis: Mosby.

Dickhut, H. W. (1987). *The executive resume handbook.* New York: Prentice-Hall.

Doak, C., Doak, L., & Root, J. (1985). *Teaching patients with low literacy skills.* Philadelphia: J. B. Lippincott.

Doehring, D. G. (1988). *Research strategies in human communication disorders.* Boston: College-Hill Press.

Dorenberg, N. (1976). The parent of a team member. *The art and science of parenting the disabled child.* Chicago: National Easter Seal Society.

Drew, C., & Hardman, M. (1985). *Designing and conducting behavioral research.* New York: Pergamon Press.

Duchan, J. F. (1999). Views of facilitated communication: What's the point? *Language, Speech, and Hearing Services in Schools, 30,* 401–407.

Duffy, J. R. (1995). *Motor speech disorders.* St. Louis: Mosby.

Dumond, V. (1990). *The elements of nonsexist usage.* New York: Prentice Hall.

Dworkin, J., & Hartman, D. (1988). *Cases in neurogenic communication disorders.* Boston: Little, Brown.

Dworkin, J. P., & Meleca, R. J. (1997). *Vocal pathologies: Diagnosis, treatment, and case studies.* San Diego: Singular.

Education for All Handicapped Children Act of 1975, 20 U. S. C. § 1400 *et seq.*

Eichorn, P., & Yankauer, A. (1987). Do authors check their references? A survey of accuracy of references in three public health journals. *American Journal of Public Health, 77*(8), 1011–1012.

Eisenstadt, A. (1972). Weakness in clinical procedures—A parental evaluation. *Asha, 14*(1), 7–9.

Elbow, P. (1998). *Writing with power: Techniques for mastering the writing process.* New York: Oxford University Press.

Emerick, L., & Haynes, W. (1986). *Diagnosis and evaluation in speech pathology.* Englewood Cliffs, NJ: Prentice Hall.

Evans, J., Nadjari, H., & Burchell, S. (1990). Quotational and reference accuracy in surgical journals: A continuing peer review problem. *Journal of the American Medical Association, 263*(10), 1353–1354.

Eysenbach, G., & Diepsen, T. L. (1998). Towards quality management of medical information on the Internet: Evaluation, labeling, and filters of information. *British Medical Journal, 317,* 1496–1502.

Fagan, E. (n.d.). *Journal clubs: An effective, convenient way to continue your life long learning.* Rockville, MD: American Speech-Language-Hearing Association.

Family Educational Rights and Privacy Act of 1974, 20 U.S.C. § 1232 *et seq.*

Farmer, J. (1989). Clinical literacy. In S. Farmer & J. Farmer (Eds.), *Supervision in communication disorders* (pp. 229–249). Columbus, OH: Merrill.

Farmer, S. (1989). Communication competence. In S. Farmer & J. Farmer (Eds.), *Supervision in communication disorders* (pp. 96–146). Columbus, OH: Merrill.

Findley, T. (1989). Research in physical medicine and rehabilitation: How to ask the question. *American Journal of Physical Medicine and Rehabilitation, 68,* 26–31.

Findley, T. W. (1990). Research in physical medicine and rehabilitation. IX: Primary data analysis. *American Journal of Physical Medicine and Rehabilitation, 69*(4), 209–218.

Findley, T. W. (1991). Research in physical medicine and rehabilitation. II: The conceptual review of the literature or how to read more articles than you ever want to see in your entire life. *American Journal of Physical Medicine and Rehabilitation, 70*(1), 517–522.

Findley, T., & Daum, M. (1989). Research in physical medicine and rehabilitation: The chart review on how to use clinical data for exploratory retrospective studies. *American Journal of Physical Medicine and Rehabilitation, 68,* 150–157.

Fink, A. (1998). *Conducting research literature reviews.* Thousand Oaks, CA: Sage.

Fishbein, M. (1950). *Medical writing: The technic and the art.* Philadelphia: The Blakiston Co.

Fitzpatrick, J., Secrist, J., & Wright, D. J. (1998). *Secrets for a successful dissertation.* Thousand Oaks, CA: Sage.

Flower, R. (1984). *Delivery of speech–language pathology and audiology services.* Baltimore: Williams and Wilkins.

Flynn, M. C., Parsons, C. L., & Shipp, L. (1999, November). Development of an interactive computerized report writer for speech–language pathology students. *Asha 21,* 1–3.

Foreman, M., & Kirchoff, K. (1987). Accuracy of references in nursing journals. *Research in Nursing and Health, 10,* 177–183.

Forscher, R., & Wertz, R. (1970). Organizing the scientific paper. *Asha, 32*(1), 39–40.

Fournier, M., & Spin, J. (1999). *Encyclopedia of job-winning resumes.* Ridgefield, CA: Round Lake Publishing.

Fowler, H. (1980). *The Little, Brown handbook.* Boston: Little, Brown.

Frattali, C. M. (1992). Peer review: Looking over your own shoulder. *Hearsay, 7*(11), 25–29.

Frattali, C. M. (1994). Quality improvement. In R. Lubinski & C. M. Frattali (Eds.), *Professional issues in speech–language pathology and audiology* (pp. 246–257). San Diego: Singular.

Frattali, C. M. (1998). Measuring modality-specific behaviors, functional abilities, and quality of life. In C. M. Frattali (Ed.), *Measuring outcomes in speech–language pathology* (pp. 55–88). New York: Thieme.

Frattali, C., & Lynch, C. (1989). Functional assessment: Current issues and future challenges. *Asha, 31*(4), 70–74.

Friel-Patti, S. (1999). Clinical decision-making in the assessment and intervention of central auditory processing disorders. *Language, Speech, and Hearing Services in Schools, 30,* 345–352.

Friske, R. (1990). *Guide to concise writing.* New York: Webster's New World.

Fuchs, L. S., & Fuchs, D. (1993). Writing research for publication: Recommendations for new authors. *Remedial and Special Education, 14*(3), 35–46.

Funk, C. J. (1998, August 3). How reliable is medical data on the World Wide Web? *Advance for Speech–Language Pathologists,* pp. 26–27.

Gardner, M. J., Mechin, D., & Campbell, M. J. (1986). Use of checklists in assessing the statistical content of medical studies. *British Medical Journal, 292,* 810–812.

Gefuert, C. (1985). *The confident writer.* New York: Norton.

Gibaldi, J., & Achtert, W. (1984). *MLA handbook for writers of research papers.* New York: Modern Language Association of America.

Gierut, J. A. (1998). Treatment efficacy: Functional phonological disorders in children. *Journal of Speech, Language, and Hearing Research, 41*(1), S85–S100.

Gillam, R. B. (1999). Computer-assisted language intervention using fast ForWord®: Theoretical and empirical considerations for clinical decision-making. *Language, Speech, and Hearing Services in Schools, 30*, 363–370.

Girder, E. R. (1996). *Evaluating research articles*. Thousand Oaks, CA: Sage.

Goldberg, R., Newton, E., Cameron, J., Jacobson, R., Char, L., Buket, W. R., & Rakab, A. (1993). References accuracy in the emergency medicine literature. *Annuals of Emergency Medicine, 22*(9), 1450–1454.

Gordon-Salant, S. (1998). Editors page: Summary publications statistics for 1997. *Journal of Speech, Language and Hearing Research, 41*, 1225–1226.

Grabois, M., & Fuhrer, M. (1988). Psychiatrists' views on research. *American Journal of Physical Medicine and Rehabilitation, 67*, 171–174.

Grapp, G. J., & Lewis, A. (1998). *How to write letter resumes*. Happase, NY: Barrons.

Green, W. (1986). Professional standards and ethics. In R. McLaughlin (Ed.), *Speech–language pathology and audiology: Issues and management* (pp. 135–159). New York: Grune and Stratton.

Greenberg, L., & Jewett, L. (1987). The case presentation: Teaching medical students writing and communication skills. *Medical Teacher, 9*(3), 281–284.

Griffer, M. R. (1999). Is sensory integration effective for children with language-learning disorders: A critical review of the evidence. *Language, Speech, and Hearing Services in Schools, 30*, 393–400.

Guyatt, G. H., Naylor, C. D., Juniper, E., Hayland, D. K., Jaeschka, R., & Cook, D. J. (1997). User's guide to the medical literature: XI. How to use articles about health-related quality of life. *Journal of the American Medical Association, 2*(15), 1232–1237.

Guyatt, G. H., Sackett, D. L., & Cook, D. J. (1994). Users' guides to the medical literature: II. How to use an article about therapy or prevention. B. What were the results and will they help me in caring for my patients? *Journal of the American Medical Association, 271*(1), 59–63.

Hamre, C. (1972). Research and clinical practice: A unifying model. *Asha, 14*(10), 542–545.

Hanson, M. (1979). The diagnostic report. In B. Hutchinson, M. Hanson, & M. Mecham (Eds.), *Diagnostic handbook of speech pathology* (pp. 30–53). Baltimore: Williams and Wilkins.

Harris, H. F. (1996). Elective mutism: A tutorial. *Language, Speech, and Hearing Services in Schools, 27*, 10–15.

Harrison, M. K. (1998). State initiations in outcomes measurement. In C. M. Frattali (Ed.), *Measuring outcomes in speech–language pathology* (pp. 514–526). New York: Thieme.

Haynes, R. B., Mulrow, C. D., Huth, E. J., Altman, D. G., & Gardner, M. J. (1996). More informative abstracts revisited. *Cleft Palate–Craniofacial Journal, 33*(1), 1–9.

Haynes, W., & Hartman, D. (1975). The agony of report writing: A new look at an old problem. *Journal of the National Student Speech Hearing Association, 1*, 7–15.

Haynes, W. O., & Pindzola, R. H. (1998). *Diagnosis and evaluation in speech pathology*. Needham Heights, MA: Allyn & Bacon.

Hays, L. H. (2000). Guide to clinical practice in the acute hospital setting. *Contemporary Issues in Communication Sciences and Disorders, 27*, 14–34.

Hegde, M. N. (1991). *Singular manual of textbook preparation*. San Diego: Singular.

Hegde, M. N. (1994). *Clinical research in communicative disorders*. Austin, TX: PRO-ED.

Hegde, M. N. (1998). *A coursebook on scientific and professional writing for speech–language pathology*. San Diego: Singular.

Hegde, M. N., & Davis, D. (1995). *Clinical methods in speech–language pathology*. San Diego: Singular.

Hegde, M. N., & Davis, D. (1999). *Clinical method and practicum in speech–language pathology*. San Diego: Singular.

Heineman, A., & Willis, H. (1988). *Writing term papers*. Orlando, FL: Harcourt, Brace & Jovanovich.

Helm-Estabrooks, N., & Aten, J. (1989). *Difficult diagnosis in adult communication disorders*. Boston: College-Hill.

Henson, K. T. (1999). *Writing for professional publication: Keys to academic and business success*. Needham Heights, MA: Allyn & Bacon.

Higdon, L., & Friel–Patti, S. (1987). *What, why, how to publish*. Paper presented to the Texas Speech-Language-Hearing Association, Houston.

Hinchcliff, K. W., Bruce, J. J., Powers, J. D., & Kipp, M. L. (1993). Accuracy of references and quotations in veterinary journals. *Journal of the American Veterinary Medicine Association, 202*(3), 397–400.

Holland, A. L. (1980). *Communicative abilities in daily living*. Austin, TX: PRO-ED.

Holland, A. L., Fromm, D. S., DeRuyter, F., & Stein, M. (1996). Treatment efficacy: Aphasia. *Journal of Speech and Hearing Research, 39*(5), S27–S36.

Holm, V., & McCartin, R. (1978). Interdisciplinary child development team: Team issues and training in interdisciplinariness. In K. Allen, V. Holm, & R. Schiefelbusch (Eds.), *Early intervention: A team approach* (pp. 97–102). Baltimore: University Park Press.

Hoolsema, E. M. (1999, May 3). Working and living with PPS. *Advance for Speech–Language Pathologists and Audiologists, 9*(18), 20–22.

Hunter, D., & Kuh, G. (1987). The "write wing": Characteristics of prolific contributors to the higher education literature. *Journal of Higher Education, 58*, 443–461.

Huth, E. (1990). *How to write and publish papers in the medical sciences*. Baltimore: Williams and Wilkins.

Hyman, R. (1995). How to critique a published article. *Psychological Bulletin, 118*(2), 178–182.

Individuals with Disabilities Education Act of 1990, 20 U.S.C. § 1400 *et seq*.

Isaac, S., & Michael, W. B. (1987). *Handbook in research and evaluation*. San Diego: Edits Publishers.

Iskowitz, M. (1999, November 15). Coding conundrum: Reimbursement varies from state to state and from one program to another. *Advance for Speech–Language Pathologists and Audiologists, 9*(46), 11, 13, 17.

Jones, S. (1976). Professional ethics. *Journal of the National Student Speech-Language-Hearing Association, 2*, 27–31.

Justice, A. C., Berlin, J. A., Fletcher, S. W., Fletcher, R. H., & Goodman, S. N. (1994). Do readers and peer reviewers agree on manuscript quality? *Journal of the American Medical Association, 272*, 117–119.

Kamhi, A. (1984). Problem solving in child language disorders: The clinician as clinical scientist. *Language, Speech, and Hearing Services in Schools, 15*(4), 226–234.

Kamhi, A. G. (1995). Research to prevention: Define, develop, and maintain clinical expertise. *Language, Speech, and Hearing Services in Schools, 26*(4), 353–356.

Kassirer, J. P., & Campion, E. W. (1994). Peer review: Crude and understudied, but indispensable. *Journal of the American Medical Association, 272*(2), 96–97.

Kay, A. (1997). *Resumes that will get you the job you want*. Cincinnati, OH: Better Way Books.

Keith, R. W. (1999). Clinical issues in central auditory processing disorders. *Language, Speech, and Hearing Services in Schools, 30*(4), 339–344.

Keith–Spiegel, P., Wittig, A. F., Perkins, D. W., Balogh, D. W., & Whitley, B. E. (1993). *The ethics of teaching*. Muncie, IN: Ball State University.

Kemp, R. J., Roeser, R. J., Pearson, D. W., & Ballachanda, B. B. (1995). *Infection control for the professions of audiology and speech–language pathology*. Chesterfield, MO: Oaktree Products.

Kennedy, J. L. (1998). *Resumes for dummies*. Foster City, CA: Dummies Press.

Kent, L., & Chabon, S. (1980). Problem-oriented records in a university speech and hearing clinic. *Asha, 22*(3), 151–155.

Kent, R. (1983). Role of research. *ASHA Reports No. 13, Proceedings of the 1983 National Conference on Under-graduate, Graduate, and Continuing Education*, pp. 76–86.

Kent, R. D. (1996). Hearing and believing: Some limits to the auditory–perceptual assessment of speech and voice disorders. *American Journal of Speech–Language Pathology, 5*, 7–23.

Kent, R. D., & Fair, J. (1985). Clinical research: Who, where, and how. *Seminars in Speech and Language, 6*(1), 23–24.

Kerlinger, F. (1973). *Foundations of behavioral research*. New York: Holt, Rinehart, and Winston.

Kettenbach, G. (1990). *Writing SOAP notes*. Philadelphia: F. A. Davis.

Key, J., & Roland, C. (1977). Reference accuracy in articles accepted for publication in the archives of physical medicine and rehabilitation. *Archives of Physical Medicine and Rehabilitation, 58*, 136–137.

Kidder, L., & Judd, C. (1986). *Research methods in social relations*. New York: Holt, Rinehart, and Winston.

King, C. R., McGuire, D. B., Longman, A. J., & Carroll-Johnson, R. M. (1997). Peer review, authorship, ethics, and conflict of interest. *Image: Journal of Nursing Scholarship, 29*(2), 163–167.

King, R., & Berger, K. (1971). *Diagnostic assessment and counseling techniques for speech pathologists and audiologists*. Pittsburgh: Stanwix House.

Kirby, R. (1989). Excellence in rehabilitation through research. *American Journal of Physical Medicine and Rehabilitation, 68*, 43–44.

Kirsch, J. (1995). *Kirsch's handbook of published law*. Los Angeles: Acrobat Books.

Knepflar, K. (1976). *Report writing in the field of communication disorders*. Danville, IL: Interstate Printers and Publishers.

Knepflar, K. (1978). Report writing for private practitioners. In R. Battin & D. Fox (Eds.), *Private practice in audiology and speech pathology* (pp. 115–136). New York: Grune and Stratton.

Koller, D. (1986). The microcomputer and administrative activities. *Texas Journal of Audiology and Speech Pathology, 12*(1), 10–12.

Kramer, M. G., Mead, C., & Leggett, G. (1995). *Prentice-Hall handbook for writers*. Englewood Cliffs, NJ: Prentice-Hall.

Kreb, R. A., & Wolf, K. E. (1997). Successful operation in the treatment outcomes driven world of managed care. *NSSHLA Clinical Series*, pp. 1–47.

Krueger, B. (1985). Computerized reporting in a public school program. *Language, Speech, and Hearing Services in the Schools, 13*(2), 135–139.

Kuster, J. M. (1997). Internet: Ethics and the Internet. *Asha, 39*, 33.

Kuzma, J. W. (1984). *Basic statistics for the health sciences*. Mountain View, CA: Mayfield.

Landsmann, M. A. (1999, October 4). E–mail guidelines for the clinician. *Advance for Speech–Language Pathologists and Audiologists*, 42.

Laney, M. (1982). Research and evaluation in the public schools. *Language, Speech, and Hearing Services in the Schools, 13*(1), 53–56.

Larkins, P. (1987). Program evaluation system (PES): Determining quality of speech–language–hearing services. *Asha, 29*(5), 21–24.

Lass, N. J., & Pannbacker, M. (1999). *The use of malpractice data as a quality improvement tool*. Unpublished manuscript.

Laupacis, A., Wells, G., Richardson, W. S., & Tuswell, P. (1994). Users' guides to the medical literature: V. How to use an article about prognosis. *Journal of the American Medical Association, 272*(3), 234–237.

Locke, L. F., Silverman, S. J., & Spindoso, W. W. (1998). *Reading and understanding research*. Thousand Oaks, CA: Sage.

Ludlow, C. (1986). The research career ladder in human communication sciences and disorders. In R. McLaughlin (Ed.), *Speech–language pathology and audiology: Issues in management* (pp. 409–411). New York: Grune and Stratton.

Luey, B. (1987). *Handbook for academic authors*. New York: Cambridge University Press.

Lund, N. J., & Duchan, J. F. (1988). *Assessing children's language in naturalistic contexts*. Englewood Cliffs, NJ: Prentice-Hall.

Lundberg, G. D., & Williams, E. (1991). The quality of a medical article. *Journal of the American Medical Association, 265*(9), 1161–1162.

Lynch, C. (1986). Harm to the public: Is it real? *Asha, 28*(6), 25–28.

Mack, K., & Skjei, E. (1979). *Overcoming writing blocks*. Boston: Houghton Mifflin.

Macrina, F. L. (1995). *Scientific integrity*. Washington, DC: American Society for Microbiology.

Madell, J. R. (1999). Auditory integration training: One clinician's view. *Language, Speech, and Hearing Services in the Schools, 30*, 371–377.

Madsen, D. (1992). *Successful dissertations and theses*. San Francisco: Jossey-Bass.

Mahmoud, S. (1992). *Research and writing: A complete guide and handbook*. White Hall, VA: Better Way Publications.

Markert, R. J. (1989). A research methods and statistics journal club for residents. *Academic Medicine, 64*(5), 223–224.

Markman, R., Markman, P., & Waddell, M. (1994). *10 steps in writing the research paper*. Woodbarry, NY: Barron's Educational Series.

Matkin, N., Ringel, R., & Snope, T. (1983). Master report of surveys and discrepancies. *ASHA Reports No. 13, Proceedings of the 1983 National Conference on Under–graduate, Graduate, and Continuing Education*, pp. 93–105.

Mauer, D. M. (1999). Issues and applications of sensory integration theory and treatment with children with language disorders. *Language, Speech, and Hearing Services in Schools, 30*, 383–392.

Maxwell, D. L., & Satake, E. (1997). *Research and statistical methods in communication disorders*. Baltimore: Williams and Wilkins.

McCarthy, P. (1990). Self assessment inventory as quality assurance tools. *Rocky Mountain Journal of Communication Disorders, 6*, 17–19.

McCullough, C. S. (1990). Computerized assessment. In C. R. Reynolds & R. W. Kamphaus (Eds.), *Handbook of psychological and educational assessment of children: Intelligence and achievement* (pp. 723–747). New York: Guilford Press.

McLeod, P. (1988). The impact of educational interventions on the reliability of teachers' assessments of student case reports. *Medical Education, 22*, 113–117.

McLeod, S. D. (1998). The quality of medical information on the Internet. *Archives of Ophthalmology, 116*(12), 1663–1665.

Mecham, M. (1979). Testing procedures appropriate for speech pathology. In B. Hutchinson, M. Hanson, & M. Mecham (Eds.), *Diagnostic handbook of speech pathology* (pp. 54–69). Baltimore: Williams and Wilkins.

Meitus, I. (1983). Clinical report and letter writing. In I. Meitus & B. Weinberg (Eds.), *Diagnosis in speech–language pathology* (pp. 287–307). Baltimore: University Park Press.

Meltzoff, J. (1998). *Critical thinking about research*. Washington, DC: American Psychological Association.

Merson, R. M., Rolnick, M. R., & Weiner, F. (1995). *The Beaumont Outcome Software System (BOSS)*. West Bloomfield, MI: Parrott Software.

Metz, D. E. (1999). Erratum. *Journal of Speech, Language, and Hearing Research, 42*, 410.

Middleton, G. F., & Pannbacker, M. (1997). *Cleft palate and related disorders*. Bisbee, AZ: Imaginart.

Miller, C., & Swift, K. (1988). *The handbook of nonsexist writing*. New York: Harper & Row.

Miller, R., & Groher, M. (1990). *Medical speech–language pathology*. Rockville, MD: Aspen.

Moran, M., & Pentz, A. (1987). Otolaryngologists' opinions of voice therapy for vocal nodules in children. *Language, Speech, and Hearing Services in the Schools, 18*(2), 172–178.

Mulkerne, D., & Mulkerne, D. (1988). *The perfect term paper: Step by step*. New York: Doubleday.

Myers-Jennings, C. (2000). Documentation requirements for speech–language pathologists in early intervention programs. *Contemporary Issues in Communication Sciences and Disorders, 27*, 53–69.

Nation, J. E., & Aram, D. M. (1977). *Diagnosis of speech and language disorders*. St. Louis: Mosby.

Neidecker, E., & Blosser, J. (1993). *School programs in speech–language: Organization and management*. Needham Heights, MA: Allyn & Bacon.

Nelson, N. (1988). *Planning individualized speech and language intervention programs: Objectives for infants, children and adolescents*. San Antonio, TX: Psychological Corporation.

net.news. (1999, December 20). *Advance for Speech–Language Pathologists and Audiologists*, p. 23.

Nicolosi, L., Harryman, E., & Kresheck, J. (1989). *Terminology of communication disorders: Speech, language, hearing*. Baltimore: Williams and Wilkins.

Nicolosi, L., Harryman, E., & Kresheck, J. (1996). *Terminology of communication disorders: Speech, language, hearing*. Baltimore: Williams and Wilkins.

Nodar, R. (1988). Area wide grand rounds in communicative disorders: A concept borrowed from medicine. *Hearsay*, pp. 22–23.

Nova Care Inc. (1989). *Documenting functional outcome*. Paper presented to the American Speech-Language-Hearing Association, St. Louis.

Nuckles, D. B., Pope, N. N., & Adams, J. D. (1993). A survey of the accuracy of references in 10 dental journals. *Operative Dentistry, 18*(1), 28–32.

O'Conner, P. T. (1999). *Words fail me*. Orlando, FL: Harcourt Brace.

O'Connor, M., & Woodford, F. (1977). *Writing scientific papers in English*. New York: Elsevier.

O'Neil-Pirozzi, T. M. (2001). Please respect patient confidentiality. *Contemporary Issues in Communication Sciences and Disorders, 28*, 48–51.

Ottenbacher, K. J. (1995). An examination of reliability in developmental research. *Developmental and Behavioral Pediatrics, 16*(3), 177–182.

Ownby, R. (1987). *Psychological reports*. Brandon, VT: Clinical Psychological Publishing.

Paden, E. P. (1970). *A history of the American Speech and Hearing Association, 1925–1958*. Rockville, MD: American Speech-Hearing Association.

Pannbacker, M. (1975). Diagnostic report writing. *Journal of Speech and Hearing Disorders, 40*(3), 367–379.

Pannbacker, M., Middleton, G. F., & Vekovius, G. T. (1996). *Ethical practices in speech–language pathology and audiology*. San Diego: Singular.

Perkins, W. (1985). From clinical dispenser to clinical scientist. *Seminars in Speech Language, 6*, 13–22.

Peterson, H. A., & Marquardt, T. P. (1994). *Appraisal and diagnosis of speech and language disorders*. Englewood Cliffs, NJ: Prentice-Hall.

Phelps, R., & Koenigsknecht, R. (1977). Attitudes of classroom teachers, learning disabilities specialists, and school principals toward speech and language programs in public elementary schools. *Language, Speech, and Hearing Services in the Schools, 8*(1), 33–45.

Plante, E., & Vance, R. (1994). Selection of preschool language tests: A data-based approach. *Language, Speech, and Hearing Services in the Schools, 25*(1), 15–24.

Pocock, S. J., Hughes, M. D., & Lee, R. J. (1987). Statistical problems in reporting of clinical trials: A survey of three medical journals. *New England Journal of Medicine, 317*, 426–432.

Polit, D. F., & Hungler, B. P. (1991). *Nursing research: Principles and methods*. Philadelphia: Lippincott.

Portney, L. G., & Watkins, M. P. (1993). *Foundations of clinical research: Applications to practice*. Norwalk, CO: Appleton & Lange.

Probst, M. A. (1998, May 11). Protecting patient records. *Advance for Speech–Language Pathologists and Audiologists*, pp. 30–31.

Pullum, G. K. (1991). *The great Eskimo vocabulary hoax*. Chicago: The University of Chicago Press.

Ramig, L. O., & Verdolini, K. (1998). Treatment: efficacy: Voice disorders. *Journal of Speech, Language, and Hearing Research, 41*(1), S100–S116.

Rao, P. R., Blosser, J., & Huffman, N. P. (1998). Measuring consumer satisfaction. In C. M. Frattali (Ed.), *Measuring outcomes in speech–language pathology* (pp. 85–121). New York: Thieme.

Reece, R. L. (1982). Editor's notebook: Texas talk. *Minnesota Medicine, 65*(12), 729–732.

Riegelman, R. K., & Hirsch, R. P. (1989). *Studying a study and testing a test: How to read the medical literature*. Boston: Little, Brown.

Ringel, R. (1972). The clinician and the researcher: An artificial dichotomy. *Asha, 14*(7), 351–353.

Rodgers, T. H., Waguespack, G. M., Hausheen, R., Boney, S., Powers, G., Bullard, J. A., Colodzin, L., McDade, M., & Gist, K. (2000). *Professional licensure*. Poster session presented at the annual meeting of the American Speech-Language-Hearing Association, Washington, DC.

Roland, C. (1976). Thoughts about medical writing. *Anesthesia and Analgesia: Current Research, 55*(5), 717–718.

Rolnick, M. J., & Merson, R. M. (1998). Collecting, analyzing, and reporting financial outcome data. In C. M. Frattali (Ed.), *Measuring outcomes in speech–language pathology* (pp. 113–133). New York: Thieme.

Rooney, A. (1986). *Word for word*. New York: Putnam.

Roth, F. P., & Worthington, C. K. (1996). *Treatment resources manual*. San Diego: Singular.

Rudestam, K. E., & Newton, R. R. (1992). *Surviving your dissertation*. Thousand Oaks: Sage.

Ruscello, D., Lass, N., Fritz, N., & Hug, M. J. (1980). Attitudes of educators toward speech–language pathology services in rural schools. *Language, Speech, and Hearing Services in the Schools, 11*(2), 145–153.

Sanders, L. (1972). *Procedure guides for evaluation of speech and language disorders in children*. Danville, IL: Interstate Press.

Sarno, M. T. (1965). A measurement of functional communication in aphasia. *Archives of Physical Medicine and Rehabilitation, 46*, 101–107.

Sarno, M. T. (1969). *Functional communication profile*. New York: Institute of Rehabilitation Medicine, New York University Medical Center.